How to Spot a Liar

How to Read People and Spot a Liar

(A Practical Approach to Speed Learn How to Read People)

Donald Hartsfield

Published By **Phil Dawson**

Donald Hartsfield

All Rights Reserved

How to Spot a Liar: How to Read People and Spot a Liar (A Practical Approach to Speed Learn How to Read People)

ISBN   978-1-998927-67-8

Legal & Disclaimer

The information contained in this book is not designed to replace or take the place of any form of medicine or professional medical advice. The information in this book has been provided for educational & entertainment purposes only.

The information contained in this book has been compiled from sources deemed reliable, and it is accurate to the best of the Author's knowledge; however, the Author cannot guarantee its accuracy and validity and cannot be held liable for any errors or omissions. Changes are periodically made to this book. You must consult your doctor or get professional medical advice before using any of the suggested remedies, techniques, or information in this book.

Table Of Contents

Chapter 1: Reason Humans Tells Lies

We face a day by day truth such that lying has changed into a definitely ordinary event. Without a doubt, there are presently institutions having a few information checking political proclamations and enterprise deliveries to expose the creations regularly added.

It's not absolutely political figures or commercial business enterprise pioneers with a restraining infrastructure mendacity to us. Lies upward push up in loads of houses, whether or no longer or no longer it's miles the younger guy ultimate over the crushed subject he says he failed to break, or the teen contributing a story for why she have grow to be hours beyond the time downside the preceding night time time.

For a few lies, the motives are confounded. In a few times, it's far to shield the liar from being rebuffed or to shield every unique character from difficulty.

The falsehood can be to attempt not to be humiliated, to conceal what is going on, or to truly have others rethink the individual telling the lie. Such mendacity isn't always honorable, but no longer hard to realize the purpose why it takes area.

It's harder to recognize the motive why certain human beings often lie without a unmistakable cause and when the untruths are normally clean to refute. Specialists say there are exceptional motivations behind why positive human beings lie habitually.

One is that the untruth being recommended won't seem like fake to the individual telling it. Dull liars can a number of the time revel in such an extra of tension that their memory is complex.

They attempt to alleviate that tension with the aid of supplying a few issue a good way to make what is taking vicinity artwork.

For that man or woman, what became certainly stated is what they need to just accept. The man or woman mendacity can also so significantly trust the untruth need to be the reality that the falsehood will become their right fact.

Individuals who lie again and again frequently want to be in price. At the aspect while the truth of a circumstance disagrees with such control, they produce an untruth that adjusts to the story they need.

Such people may additionally additionally likewise pressure they'll no longer be seemed if fact can depart them looking ineffectively. All subjects considered, they offer an untruth that initiatives them in high-quality light, but they cannot see that thru and massive that what they supplied has no premise as a sizable rule.

It might be amazing if we would accept all that we're counseled, whether or not or no longer from that little one with the wrecked box or from that legislator at a political meeting. However, that may not arise and ultimately, each one folks need to in some instances dig specially extra profound and attempt to song down the genuine truth.

Nine Motives For Telling Lie

For what purpose in all actuality do human beings lie? Such a clean inquiry want to accompany a straightforward reaction (but does no longer, sadly). There are signs and symptoms, no matter the reality that, that a huge element humans share comparable belief procedures in lying.

The handiest method to let recognize if any character is mendacity

Numbers do not lie

My facts amassed in the course of interviews with youngsters and from polls finished with the aid of grown-usaproposes that lying takes place (to 3 degree to a constrained amount) for taken into consideration considered one of 9 reasons:

1. To strive now not to be rebuffed. This is the most customarily referenced belief for mendacity (via the usage of the 2 children and grown-ups). It's critical to take word that there have been no brilliant contrasts amongst lies knowledgeable to keep away from discipline for deliberate wrongdoing rather than an harmless mistakes.

2. To get a prize isn't always in any case proper away realistic. This is the second one maximum generally referenced idea manner, through the 2 children and grown-ups. An example of this is erroneously ensuring work insight at some stage in a potential employee assembly to assemble opportunities of recruiting.

Three. To defend someone else from being rebuffed. Similarly as with deceiving avoid individual problem, concept gadget won't change with the plan. We've visible this show up amongst colleagues, companions, family, or even with outsiders!

Four. To guard oneself from the chance of real harm. This is specific about being rebuffed, for the threat of damage is not hundreds for wrongdoing. A model might be a infant who is domestic on my own telling an interloper on the entryway that his dad is napping now and to go lower back later.

Five. To win the profound admire of others. Lying to boom your notoriety can bypass from "harmless elaborations" to improving a tale being advised to developing a completely new (artificial) person.

6. To get away an off-kilter social state of affairs. Instances of how lying can examine the equal time as propelled by way of manner of manner of this are professing to have a sitter hassle to get away a silly celebration, or completing a cellphone dialogue thru saying there may be any man or woman on the entryway.

7. To stay some distance from humiliation. The teenager who asserts the wet seat befell due to water spilling, now not from wetting her jeans, is a version if the kid did now not fear location, surely disgrace.

Eight. To keep up with safety with out telling others of that cause. For example, the couple professes to have run off due to the reality the rate of a marriage was too an prolonged manner within the crimson even as, really, they have been retaining away from the dedication to welcome their households.

Nine. To exercise manage over others with the aid of the use of using controlling the records the intention has. Broadly typified with the aid of Hitler, that is reputedly the maximum risky motive for lying.

I suspect inspirations are the use of mendacity that fall out of doors one of the over nine instructions, as an example, minor trickeries like falsehoods informed out of appropriate manners or politeness, which aren't handily subsumed with the resource of these 9 notion methods.

MORE REASONS PEOPLE DO LIE

*CAUTIOUS: The most famous justification for lying is to self-shield. There can be a authentic very last consequences or an obvious one which an individual is attempting to defend themselves in the direction of.

*MALEVOLENT: Some human beings lie purposefully to damage others thinking about the fact that they experience hurt with the aid of that man or woman. It is an approach to getting once more at someone else.

*DISSATISFACTION: In a request to attempt not to frustrate someone else or maybe themselves, an untruth may be advised. The awkward sensation of disillusionment legitimizes the trickiness.

*CONTROL: An oppressive individual continually lies to preserve with their manage. Assuming truth emerged, the manhandled should go away.

*SCARED: Sometimes absolutely faux is carried out because of the truth the man or woman feels threatened through others.

Once greater, this sensation of inadequacy is awkward to the component that they mislead cover it up.

*CONSIDERATION SEEKING: Unfortunately, some individuals lie without a doubt to face out from others. The incongruity is that the amazing majority of them do not know a way to manipulate the eye once they do get it.

*INTEREST: This is a very innocent way of behaving that some grown-united statesdo no longer outgrow. All topics considered, they lie sincerely to witness what's going to appear irrespective of what the harm it is able to purpose others.

*PREVALENT: For human beings with an exquisite self-photograph and to hold up with their predominance, they lie to reason themselves to seem trendy more attractive than others.

*COVER: Some people placed on a veil and declare to be some issue they will be now not. To hold up with their appearances, they mislead disguise any attempt to discover the actual character.

*CONTROL: Sadly, at times the entirety comes down to govern. With an quit intention to govern some one-of-a-kind person's conduct, an untruth is suggested.

*DAWDLE: Passive-forcefully staying some distance from liabilities is stalling. This falsehood is greater unobtrusive in that the individual realizes they must study thru with some issue however is intentionally putting it off.

*EXHAUSTED: Some human beings like to expose off in their lives. So they lie to paintings it up and watch the responses of others.

*SECURE: There are some lies which is probably completed to shield others. At instances, a faux being is cautioned to get a experience of ownership with things they're no longer liable for in that frame of thoughts to assist each other character.

*PROPENSITY: After a time-body and finished continually sufficient, unfortunate conduct patterns can frame. This is valid for sure untruths which may be stated time and again.

*FUN: Some humans lie as their kind of non-public diversion. For their features, mendacity is amusing due to the truth that they favor to see how others solution.

*WANT: an character who keeps that an untruth ought to be fact profoundly desires to take delivery of as authentic with their misperception.

*HURT: People who need to harm others are unsure, and lie about what their identification is and what they may be doing. This is a stylish method at some level in the abduction of others.

*COMPASSION: Similar to interest chasing, an character is trying to get sympathy from others by manner of using lying approximately a beyond or present day development.

*LETHARGIC: now and again, obviously fake reduces to an individual being slow and now not having any preference to perform the artwork, in order that they lie about it.

*DETACHMENT: If a component or hassle doesn't make a distinction to an person, they'll lie about it and now not see some factor amiss with their duplicity.

*INSIGHT: Some humans recollect their falsehood. Their affect of the fact isn't always real so in their eyes, it's far some factor however faux.

*HOIST: Individuals must beautify themselves to special people's degree of high profound top notch, robust tough going for walks thoughts-set, or perfectionistic mind, really so they deceive carry themselves.

*Dazzle: As an approach to attempting to intrigue others and purpose a advanced impact, an individual may also want to lie about what their identity is, what they've achieved, or in which they're going.

*DESIRE: When an man or woman desires what others have, they desire the element or person and lie approximately their envy.

*LIMIT: As an method to lowering the harm, mischief, or outcomes that could by means of a few approach take area, an man or woman limits reality in their untruth

*EXPAND: On the furthest side, an man or woman also can need to overstate their falsehood and exacerbate the state of affairs more than what it clearly is.

*SUPPRESS: In jogging to cover an hassle, an character have to stifle truth. This falsehood is planned.

*DENY: Not every person who does now not keep that some thing ought to exist with the aid of denying the fact is mendacity deliberately. Here and there this is inadvertent.

*STOW AWAY: An man or woman might also moreover need to cover themselves, others, or subjects and lie approximately doing as which include a technique for staying a long way from duty. This is drastically speakme completed associated with addiction-forming conduct.

Chapter 2: Signals To Notice Is Someone Telling A Lie

Instructions to Recognize the Signs That Someone Is Lying

Lying and trickiness are normal human methods of behaving. Until fairly as of overdue, there was a minimum actual research into precisely how regularly people lie. A 2004 Reader's Digest survey observed that as severa as ninety six% of individuals confess to lying to some diploma in some cases.

One public assessment allotted in 2009 studied 1,000 U.S. Grown-united statesand observed that as 60% of respondents assured that they did not lie thru any manner.

All topics being equal, the experts located that about a part of all falsehoods were cautioned with the useful resource of first-rate five% of the multitude of subjects.

The evaluation recommends that even as predominance prices may additionally moreover range, there likely exists a hint accumulating of extremely efficient liars.

A great many humans will possibly lie every occasionally. A element of these falsehoods are innocent exaggerations deliberate to protect every other man or woman's sentiments ("No, that shirt does now not make you look fats!"). In outstanding instances, those falsehoods can be extensively extra right (like mendacity on a resume) or hundreds greater vile (concealing wrongdoing).

Lying Can Be Hard to Detect

Individuals are shockingly horrible at spotting lies. One evaluation, for example, determined that human beings have been sincerely ready to precisely distinguish mendacity 54% of the time in a lab placing — scarcely notable at the equal time as figuring in a half of reputation fee via unadulterated possibility on my own.

Conduct contrasts amongst expert and lying people are difficult to segregate and quantify. Specialists have endeavored to discover numerous techniques to distinguishing lies. While there won't be a sincere indication that any character is dishonest (like Pinocchio's nose), scientists have tracked down more than one supportive markers.

In the same manner as diverse matters, but, identifying a falsehood regularly boils right all the way down to a sure some issue — taking note of your intestine emotions. By information what signs and symptoms and signs and symptoms and signs and symptoms must precisely choose out an untruth and figuring out a manner to word your stomach responses, you can have the selection to turn out to be better at spotting lies.

INDICATIONS OF LYING

Analysts have used research on non-verbal communique and misdirection to assist people in policing and spotting fact and untruths. Specialists at UCLA directed examinations concerning the trouble similarly to breaking down 60 examinations on duplicity to foster pointers and put together for policing. The effects in their exploration have been allocated in the American Journal of Forensic Psychiatry.

Warnings That Someone May Be Lying

A couple of the functionality warnings the scientists diagnosed that might monitor that humans are underhanded embody:

Being ambiguous; presenting no longer many subtleties

Rehashing inquiries before responding to them

Talking in sentence quantities

Neglecting to offer specific subtleties even as a tale is tested

Prepping methods of behaving, as an example, gambling with hair or squeezing hands, identifying trickiness is in no way clean, best schooling can paintings on an man or woman's capability to distinguish lies:

"Without steering, many humans discern they could distinguish misdirection, however, their insights are beside the point to their real potential. Speedy, insufficient instructional meetings lead people to over-examine and to do greater terrible things than within the occasion that they go together with their belly responses.

METHODS FOR IDENTIFYING LYING

If you think that any man or woman probable won't be coming smooth, there are multiple methodologies you could employ that could help with recognizing truth from fiction.

Try now not to Rely on Body Language Alone

With regards to spotting lies, people often middle spherical non-verbal communication "tells," or inconspicuous bodily and social symptoms and signs that find out misdirection. While non-verbal communique symptoms and symptoms and signs and symptoms can once in a while allude to double-dealing, studies proposes that many predicted approaches of behaving are not normally related with lying.

Scientist Howard Ehrlichman, a clinician who has been targeting eye development because the 1970s, has placed that eye improvement does no longer recommend lying via any stretch of the imagination. He recommends that moving eyes recommend that an man or woman is questioning, or all the greater definitively, that the man or woman is attending to their drawn-out reminiscence.

Different examinations have validated that at the same time as person signs and strategies of behaving are useful marks of trickery, a part of those most usually associated with mendacity (like eye developments) are some of the most terrible predictors. So at the same time as non-verbal verbal exchange can be a treasured gadget in the discovery of untruths, the secret's to realize which symptoms and symptoms and symptoms and signs to cognizance on.

Center Around the Right Signals

One meta-examination determined that on the equal time as people do often depend on widespread prompts for figuring out lies, the hassle need to lie with the incapacity of these signs as duplicity markers in any case.

Probably the most reliable trickery turns on that individuals truely do cognizance on embody:

Being ambiguous: If the speaker appears to deliberately leave out huge subtleties, it may thoroughly be due to the fact they'll be mendacity.

Vocal vulnerability: If the individual seems to be unsure or shaky, they're certain to be apparent as an untruth.

Detachment: Shrugging, absence of articulation, and an exhausted stance can be signs and symptoms of mendacity due to the fact the individual is attempting to attempt now not to hold emotions and capability tells.

Overthinking: If the individual is with the aid of all money owed thinking too difficult to even undergo in thoughts filling in the subtleties of the story, it very well can be due to the truth they may be deluding you.

The instance proper here is that at the same time as non-verbal verbal exchange is probably useful, focusing on the proper indicators is huge. Nonetheless, some experts advise that relying too vigorously on unique symptoms and symptoms and signs and symptoms may also disable the capability to recognize lies.

Request that they Tell Their Story in Reverse

Lie area have to be visible as an uninvolved interplay. Individuals would possibly assume they're able to in reality examine the ability liar's non-verbal conversation and appearance to come across self-evident "tells." In adopting a extra dynamic approach for uncovering lies, you could yield advanced results.

Some exam has encouraged that requesting that human beings document their bills backward request in place of sequential request can growth the precision of untruth popularity. Verbal and non-verbal activates that recognize mendacity and truth-telling may also come to be greater clean as highbrow burden increases.

Lying is more intellectually burdening than coming smooth. On the off threat which you add notably more intellectual intricacy, behavior turns on may additionally end up greater obvious.

In addition to the reality that telling is false and greater intellectually soliciting for, liars generally observe appreciably extra mental electricity inside the direction of observing their techniques of behaving and assessing the reactions of others. They are concerned about their validity and ensuring that others trust their payments. This calls for an entire lot of exertion, so if you toss in a difficult mission (like concerning their tale in switch request), breaks inside the tale and exclusive behavior tips should turn out to be more truthful to find out.

In one assessment, 80 fake suspects each came easy or lied approximately an prepared occasion. A a part of the human beings were approached to document their money owed backward request while others mentioned their money owed in sequential requests. The experts located that the communicate request interviews exposed extra social guidelines to double-dealing.

In a subsequent trial, fifty 5 police officers watched taped interviews from the number one examination and have been approached to decide out who have turn out to be mendacity and who come to be now not. The exam exposed that cops were higher at recognizing lies within the opposite request interviews than they were inside the sequential conferences.

Pay Attention To Your Gut Feelings

Your quick belly responses can be extra true than any cognizant untruth place you could challenge. In one look at, experts had seventy people watch recordings of meetings with mock wrongdoing suspects. Some of these suspects had taken a $a hundred dollar from off a shelf while others had now not, but the suspects have been all informed to permit the questioner apprehend that that that they'd no longer taken the coins.

Like past examinations, the people could not reliably understand lies, in truth precisely distinguishing the liars forty 3% of the time and fact tellers 48% of the time.

However, the analysts moreover used understood social response time tests to evaluate the people' greater programmed and oblivious reactions to the suspects. What they determined changed into that the topics had been positive to unwittingly relate words like "deceptive" and "underhanded" with the suspects which have been lying. They were moreover fantastic to verifiably associate phrases like "giant" and "real" with reality tellers.

The outcomes suggest that people may want to possibly have an oblivious, instinctive belief concerning whether or not or now not someone is lying.

So assuming our stomach responses can be more precise, why are people worse at spotting untruthfulness? Cognizant reactions may additionally want to disrupt our programmed affiliations. Rather than relying on our senses, people middle throughout the cliché processes of behaving that they often associate with mendacity, as an instance, squirming and lack of eye-to-eye connection. Overemphasizing techniques of behaving that problematically count on double-dealings makes it more hard to understand reality and falsehoods.

There isn't any trendy, reliable sign that any person is lying. Each of the symptoms, methods of behaving, and suggestions that scientists have related to mendacity are virtually quantities of information that would locate whether or not or no longer an character is straightforward.

Whenever you are attempting to test the veracity of a completely unique tale, prevent taking a gander on the unoriginal "lying signs and signs and symptoms" and figure out the way to recognize greater unpretentious methods of behaving that may be related to trickiness. At the problem even as important, adopt a more dynamic approach with the beneficial resource of along with pressure and make lying all of the more intellectually burdening thru inquiring for that the speaker relate the story in transfer request.

At last, and perhaps, in particular, be privy to your intestine feelings. You ought to have a truely herbal feeling of trustworthiness versus deceitfulness. Figure out the manner to be conscious the ones premonitions.

TOP 10 SIGNS THAT SOMEONE IS LYING

Did you have any idea that exceptional fifty four% of falsehoods may be precisely spotted? Likewise, outgoing human beings will generally lie more than self observers, as indicated with the aid of Vanessa Van Edwards, writer of the overall public wreck hit e-book Captivate and pioneer and lead examiner of the Science of People.

As in step with her exploration, a few issue like 82% of untruths goes undetected, which drove her to foster a path in lie identification named "How to Be a Human Lie Detector." The numbers show that this sort of path might be a clever project: in a evaluate named "Predominance of Lying in America," absolutely six out of ten Americans professed to return back easy constantly.

With numbers like the ones, one u . S . A ., no matter whether or now not or no longer having sworn to inform the fact, might not be fairly dependable.

Fortunately, regardless of the fact that typically, 50% of the populace vows to be coming easy, there are some special strategies people can expand their truth expertise capabilities to guard themselves from close to domestic and financial smash.

While lie discovery courses are essential for eye-to-eye connections, the untruths that cause the maximum monetary harm within the 21st century occur over broadcast communications. As indicated thru USA.Gov, correspondence channels like smartphone, e-mail, message, online classifieds, or digital amusement are implemented to trick or undermine individuals to provide out their records or cash.

Exactly how masses well-deserved cash has been misplaced through human beings beneath coercion? In 2018, trick casualties unique losing $1.Forty eight billion in extortion — a lovely boom of 38% from 2017, as in step with the Federal Trade Commission (FTC).

What's more, the casualties are not quality beneficiaries; in that body of mind, in their 20s located dropping a normal of $4 hundred contrasted with $751 for humans in their 70s. That massive variety dramatically progressed for individuals of their 80s who out of place a everyday of $1,seven hundred throughout the same time.

It cannot be expressed frequently enough: to protect your financial and individual assets from liars, in no way beneath any condition deliver out your facts or pass coins thru wire to everyone you have no concept about.

Whether you are coping with bogus net-based dangers or exploitative individuals misleading your face, this has but to be addressed: what are the signs and symptoms and signs and symptoms that someone is lying? As regular with Vanessa Van Edwards, this is quite possibly the earliest enhance in getting snug with how every body commonly acts.

This is the approach worried in laying out a sample, which she characterizes as "How each person acts at the same time as they may be below ordinary, innocent events, how everybody seems while they're coming easy."

All in all, it can be difficult to tell at the same time as someone is mendacity if you do not have the foggiest concept of how they act even as they may be coming smooth, which highlights the significance of laying out entrust with someone in advance than you percent individual statistics. For example, it is in each case superb to call your economic organization straightforwardly and recognize who you're speaking with as opposed to believing each person who calls aimlessly or locations an professional-looking letter via the positioned up office professing to be a financial group worker.

Then yet again, at the off risk which you recognise any individual and regard yourself as considering whether or not you are being informed every bit of relevant information or a deceptive declaration, here's a generation-supported rundown of the pinnacle

1. A CHANGE IN SPEECH PATTERNS

One indication anyone may not be telling each little little bit of applicable facts is unpredictable discourse. As regular with Gregg mccrary, a retired FBI crook profiler, an person's voice or quirks of speakme may also exchange after they lie, as investigated by means of Real Simple.

Mccrary first takes the method of recognizing an individual's normal discourse examples and idiosyncrasies thru asking run-of-the-mill, direct inquiries, for instance, what their call is or wherein they live. This permits him to look any progressions in speakme or attributes whilst he significantly assessments inquisitive inquiries.

2. THE USE OF NON-CONGRUENT GESTURES

If an character says OK however shakes their head no, it'd show off that they'll be no longer coming clean. As Dr. Ellen Hendriksen, a systematic clinician at Boston University's Center for Anxiety and Related Disorders, brings up in Scientific American, non-consistent motions are tendencies in the frame that don't healthy the phrases an man or woman says, and the signs and symptoms are fact tellers. According to Hendricksen's version, if any man or woman, "manifestly i'll assist out with the exam" and offers a touch head shake, it's far plausible they won't tell each little bit of applicable information and best reality.

3. NOT SAYING ENOUGH

While truth-telling observers depict what they found and are inquired: "Is there a few aspect else?" greater subtleties are exposed. In any case, at the same time as liars are approached to move past their pre-organized memories, no longer many to nobody in every of a type subtleties are advertised.

Scientists stated in the American Psychological Association (APA) allude to those individuals as "liars who bamboozle through exclusion," who, at the same time as asked to cope with inquiries or provide greater subtleties, regularly provide not precisely the ones coming clean.

This can be measured via records of calls, witness proclamations, or saw by means of using a shortfall of expressive phrases in a talk.

Another manner scientists take a look at the truth of the trouble is through requesting that people inform sports in contrary. Truth-tellers will maintain up with similar debts at the same time as presenting greater subtleties, whilst liars frequently get involved and make an exchange story at the same time as now not collectively with subtlety to the primary.

Four. CROSSING THE LINE

On the alternative facet, scientists from Harvard Business School confirmed that liars attempting to trick exaggerate with an excessive form of phrases. Since one of these liar may want to probable make up topics as they circulate, they'll likewise generally upload exorbitant element to steer themselves or others of what they're talking approximately. They can also additionally likewise decorate with terms that an person coming clean could not don't forget including.

Other phonetic signs uncovered in this take a look at display that liars will normally utilize extra foulness and 1/three-man or woman pronouns (e.G., he, she, and they) to reduce most, if no longer all, connection with any first-man or woman (e.G., I, my, mine) association.

5. AN UNUSUAL RISE OR FALL IN VOCAL

TONE

In a similar APA article, a brilliant issue is raised spherical tradition, setting, and correspondence regarding recognizing lies.

Dr. David Matsumoto, a teacher of thoughts technological expertise at San Francisco State University and CEO of Humintell, a counseling employer that trains people to peruse human emotions, stresses that experts need to consider social inclination on the identical time as identifying whether or no longer someone is mendacity or no longer. For instance, his falsehood reputation research located that Chinese members will extra often than no longer speak with a better vocal pitch whilst lying.

In direct difference, Hispanic exam individuals talked with a lower vocal pitch whilst mendacity.

This exam demonstrates the manner that non-verbal activates for lying may be associated with social contrasts, which need to be concept approximately in preference to judging simply from one's social convictions.

6. BEARING OF THEIR EYES

Much has been stated almost about honesty and eye-to-eye connection. A normally held social self assure within the United States is: that if an man or woman isn't visually connecting, they're no longer coming clean, even though, in specific societies, eye-to-eye connection may be seemed as cheating in a given setting.

A assessment named "The Eyes Don't Have It," distributed in 2012 in Plos One, uncovered the concept that humans appearance left or proper on the identical time as mendacity.

Nonetheless, an examination achieved in 2015 via way of the University of Michigan and highlighted in Time Magazine confirmed that 70% of people in a hundred and twenty media cuts lied whilst preserving in touch.

7. COVERING THEIR MOUTH OR EYES

Many people need to cover a falsehood or stow far from their response to it, which is probably the reason they located their palms over their eyes or mouths at the same time as letting a misrepresentation out. As in step with previous CIA officers in their ebook Spy the Lie, others would likely try and close their eyes at the same time as mendacity, as precise in Parade Magazine. This can be especially apparent even as the mild of an inquiry does no longer want a ton of meditated image.

8. UNNECESSARY FIDGETING

Ponder what a youngster does even as asked wherein the closing address went. They may additionally additionally lick their lips, take a gander at their nails, or perhaps shake their arms — and in a while inform a chief humdinger of a falsehood.

What's taking place is that their uneasiness response has kicked in, making blood be removed from their limits. They might be unknowingly seeking to quiet that anxiety response or possibly soar-start the tool back to their limits, all of that could highlight apprehension about lying.

9. BLAME SHIFTING (LITERAL OR FIGURATIVE)

The demonstration of pointing at or in the direction of some different person or aspect, with motions or phrases, may additionally flag a reliable yearning to eliminate a interest from an man or woman and word fault onto each different person, as indicated by means of Business Insider.

Knowing whether that man or woman commonly indicators or finger focuses often may be a beneficial desired. In any case, assuming any man or woman talks in a planned disposition in desire to an unfriendly one which includes blame-transferring, this forceful switch would likely display all of us is mendacity.

10. SELF-IDENTIFYING AS A "GREAT LIAR"

Maybe the least worrying approach for detecting a liar is to permit them to do it for you. In a evaluation named "Falsehood pervasiveness, lie tendencies and techniques of self-precise extremely good liars," studies dispensed in 2019 in Plos One showed that the oldsters that are identified as "superb liars" are a more quantity of a respectable marker than lie finder exams.

That's what this check showed: "first rate liars" commonly lied to friends and partners face to face and zeroed in on recounting simple and clean testimonies. This examination's simple hobby factor is that assuming anybody gloats approximately being a top notch liar, they don't have any faith in them.

THE BOTTOM LINE: IS IT POSSIBLE TO TELL IF SOMEONE IS LYING?

While criminology specialists are prepared to gain structures to awaken fact from fiction, you do not want to be a crook investigator or very private a falsehood locator gadget to recognize at the same time as any person may additionally lie eye to eye, thru cellular telephone, or in an e mail or message.

Commonly, fact can be emotional and individual factors of view can slant what is actual and not proper. The systems used to recognize an untruth can in some instances be confounding or in any event, clashing. To this element, a evaluation distributed in the British Psychological Society showed that people with improved degrees of the potential to understand people on a profound stage might also need to peruse people properly but enjoy trouble finding out whether or not or not an character tale is underhanded or no longer.

And maintaining in thoughts that the signs and symptoms and signs recorded above rely on quantitative (showed via mathematical records) and subjective (affirmed by using the use of portrayal) research, no unmarried technique need to be finished on my own as a figuring out variable for purchasing any man or woman is faux for individual or policing. Analysts supply their all to configuration concentrates on that confine particular evidence, but, every condition is novel and should be handled carefully relying upon conditions.

Chapter 3: Decoding Body Language

"The body can't lie." Learning to peruse the unobtrusive symptoms and symptoms that let us understand even as an man or woman is lying is a large benefit in our non-public and enterprise organization connections, she says, at the side of, "Ensure you're focusing, or you may pay with torment."

Step through step instructions to Confront a Liar

If you accept as true with you studied any person is lying, pose more inquiries. Take an instance from the prison cross-examinations you note on TV. Pointed inquiries concerning the complex "realities" may also need to reason them to construct more lies — however presently you can peruse their non-verbal communique to hit upon indicators of trickiness. When squeezed further, the priority could harm down and are available easy with you

1. Crisscrossed Words and Body Language

In our manner of lifestyles, stirring one's head in some unspecified time in the future of implies sincerely, and element to aspect manner no. On the off threat that any man or woman is announcing, "No, I did no longer make it take place," but their head is shaking indeed, they maximum likely got it performed. "Individuals subliminally emphasize subjects with their heads continuously," says Brown, and the top is more reliable than the mouth.

For models, watch video clasps of excessive-profile figures denying right allegations — all on the same time as shaking their heads positive: President Bill Clinton demanding he didn't have sexual members of the family with Monica Lewinsky; jonbenét Ramsey's dad announcing he did no longer murder his little girl; and Patriots quarterback Tom Brady stated he did not empty the football.

2. Huge, Bold, and Bogus

Assuming every body hinders others on occasion, occupies bunches of room with their arm indicators and stance, and is stone faced on the equal time as talking, be considerably attentive. These developments often can discover a rehearsed misrepresentation. (Watch the records and take a look at!)

3. Multiplying Down on Deception

Individuals who're most unrestrained in their disavowals or particular fake proclamations are in all likelihood going to be blameworthy. "The ones who are taking a stab at seeming as in spite of the reality that the hero are human beings we need to be careful about," says Brown, who, as a previous professional motorbike owner, counts Lance Armstrong — and severa ongoing political figures — some of the offenders.

4. Lips Don't Lie

Collapsing in one's lips before talking is a warning. "At the factor while people' lips vanish, they will be retaining down statistics," said Brown. "The following factor that emerges from their mouth is both a misleading assertion or a falsehood."

Hand protective mouth shows a falsehood

These are feature-looking techniques of overlaying the mouth. At the thing when posed a proper away inquiry, the following element said is normally bogus.

5. A Hand-to-Mouth Giveaway

Notice even as anybody covers their mouth with their hand, even incompletely. It seems ordinary however often shows that the subsequent detail they're pronouncing is bogus. On the off chance that you inquire, "For what motive did you go away your very last function?" and their hand comes as a lot as their mouth as they forestall all of sudden and afterward say, "I grew out of the area," they may be preserving down facts.

To draw out fact, you could answer: "It looks as if you have were given extra to say. Need to amplify that?"

6. Be Attuned to Tone

Manner of speakme is likely the satisfactory sign of double-dealing. A robust "persuading" tone regularly demonstrates duplicity, on the same time as a gentler "conveying" tone can endorse any character is telling a fractional truth and not the complete story.

7. Notice the Jitters

Assuming all of us turns into nervous, that could display double-dealing. Our ft provide us the texture to break out what is going on, and while our cerebrums permit us to apprehend we can't try this, a touch moving setup may be the outcome

8. Search for Inconsistencies

Individuals have run-of-the-mill designs for his or her varieties of non-verbal communique and manner of talking. Assuming someone's non-verbal communication is bizarre for that individual, take a look at.

9. Doubt a Delay

Assuming any man or woman stands through over 5 seconds to reply to an inquiry, that may be a very respectable indication of double-dealing.

10. Indeed or No Isn't Maybe

I suspect as masses,`"I do now not keep in mind" or "seemingly" are suspect solutions to any sure-or-no inquiry.

11. Spy Anxious Eyes

"At the issue whilst you observe the whites of human beings' eyes, meaning dread, On the off hazard that any character's eyes dart spherical after they've posed an inquiry — transferring up, down, and issue-to-issue — they're hesitant to provide a dependable reaction.

Grin within the eyes is actual

Notice the grin on the left consisting of the eyes. That is a real grin.

12. Truth is inside the Crow's Feet

Certified grins commonly include the eyes. Search for crow's toes. For example, if a organization touch says, "this is an undertaking we're amped up for" and you see those little kinks attaining out from their eyes towards their sanctuaries, their delight is certifiable. If you do not see crow's feet, be cautious: Confidence is being exaggerated.

13. Observe the Blink Rate

On the off danger that any individual's eyes flicker all the extra fast at the identical time as tending to a selected scenario or responding to precise inquiries, this is

A demonstration of hysteria, which regularly harmonizes with a falsehood.

Assuming there has been an illustration that indicated to others that that character is mendacity, they might now not make it take location. Be that as it could, there isn't always one.

Nobody piece of nonverbal correspondence can permit us to understand if absolutely everyone is misdirecting us or clearly lying. Individuals would love untruths assuming that there had been.

The number one manner we can decide whether or not any man or woman is deceiving us is through using trying to find caution symptoms and signs and symptoms of trickiness. We need to parent out the way to peruse seems, frame traits, tone, and rhythm of voice in advance than we are capable of determine a preference assuming that that man or woman is deceiving us.

Spotting double-dealing requires facts what conduct a liar will display as they make up their tale.

It's a few factor however a few aspect clean to get lies.

Why Words Are Less Important Than You Think

Looks, voice intonation, act, and respiratory propensities are exceedingly huge factors to remember at the equal time as perusing non-verbal conversation.

These numerous assets also can talk records all of the while and concurrently, viewing for the attention of a falsehood catcher.

It's virtually everyday that the untruth locator necessities to 0 in on areas in which there are caution symptoms of potential unscrupulousness or disparities in the announcement.

Only one out of every normal wellspring of facts in a dialogue is further sturdy. A few assets release more than others.

A high-quality many people are more focused for the duration of the maximum unreliable assets, like terms and looks which is probably effects deceived.

A have a look at has mounted that maximum liars do no longer attempt to conceal their sports and permit themselves recognize it is all inexpensive. By and large, people probably could not have the ability to achieve this regardless of whether or not or no longer they had been trying.

Individuals who falsehood try to preserve what they are stowing far from being visible through the individual they're misleading.

The folks that lie usually attempt to be greater cautious about their preference of phrases. The considerable majority studies nearly without delay in existence that humans pay interest to what is stated, so liars are in plenty of times aware about what they are saying.

Words are the incredible method for offering thinking about the fact that they're capable of convey a long way beyond some different medium. Covering greater subjects considerably quicker is a location in which terms let you succeed.

Liars will quite regularly adjust their discourse in order now not to uncover sensitive material. They do that every because they understand it is conceivable you're giving close to attention and due to the fact they realise they will be taken into consideration extra accountable.

The Face

Individuals will frequently express subjects approximately what you look like, which includes in your face. You might possibly pay interest things like they gave me a sideways look, they are searching at me, and so forth.

Individuals frequently middle round a face, some component meant to symbolize what truely makes us what our identification is. It recognizes us from others and is in many instances the primary problem we see after collecting an character

Individuals provide a excellent deal of hobby to faces. The face can display emotions and can impart how the speaker feels about what they are talking approximately.

Visually connecting is a large piece of a talk. Assuming any person's glancing towards you, it can display that they are focusing and expertise what you are saying. Yet, there are exemptions to the equal vintage: a number of the time people will grin or gesture whilst now not taking note of what you're talking about.

Liars regularly display display which additives of their phrases or non-verbal communication human beings need to zero in on more. While speaking, they will generally respond in a manner on the manner to appear like greater convincing, therefore.

It is vital to recognition on the indicators of the underhanded manner of behaving considering that words aren't generally the quality spot to look. The face is usually better for this because it friends straightforwardly with the vicinity of the mind associated with emotions and words do now not;

For example, emotions, as an instance, outrage might have an impact on our countenances automatically. Be that as it could, we are able to figure out a manner to control the ones articulations thru propensity or realistic desire.

Quite possibly the most reliable approach for sorting out whether or not or no longer or not anybody is mendacity is through their non-verbal conversation. You can confirm this thru the use of seeing if there are any progressions from their sample or conventional manner of behaving.

There is a ton of facts accessible at the net and a few vicinity else on the awesome manner to discover a liar, however, we have got blanketed the maximum famous signs and signs and symptoms and symptoms under.

The Face Can Be a Valuable Source of Information

Individuals rent their appears to speak the scope of emotions, however there may be no hazard of coming easy at the identical time as they're telling or mendacity.

Lying commonly includes sending one message and stowing away some other. This is frequently completed via displaying one face however covering every other.

At instances individuals lie and a number of the time they arrive smooth. One great method for locating out is to search for a look - a falsehood can be double-crossed thru a face that looks phony, at the identical time as any man or woman coming smooth regularly can't face up to the urge to have a few sentiments spill via.

Misleading however persuading articulations can also occur one 2nd and disguise of said articulations arise the following.

It is even possible for the felt and deceptive seems to be displayed in numerous quantities of the face indoors a solitary blended demeanor. A superb many human beings cannot understand lies thru the usage of taking a gander on the face due to the fact that they are uncertain of a way to understand bogus appears.

The legitimate, veritable articulations of feeling are added approximately through out of control facial tendencies.

It is viable to deliberately manage the face for correspondence, albeit this doesn't make correspondence any more strong.

Is Yawning A Sign Of Lying

Not a threat. Yawning without anyone else isn't demonstrative of double-dealing.

At the issue whilst every person yawns they may be taking off their mouth full-size. This makes it difficult to lie due to the fact the man or woman currently desires to move their mouth spherical to speak, that is hard to do with a significant open mouth.

Yawning is a sign of being worn-out, but, the very last results of yawning being a non-verbal verbal exchange for lying stands.

Is Blushing A Sign Of A Liar

Ordinarily, people end up flushed while they're humiliated about something. It's occasionally used to cover that they may be having an embarrassed or humiliated outlook on what has passed off. It's important at the off hazard which you spot a person becoming flushed with a chunk of facts. As ever we have to peruse in bunches to provide you a more amount of idea at the most talented technique to peruse people. If it is not too much problem, take a look at our newbie's aide on non-verbal verbal exchange... ....

Is Touching Your Face A Sign Of Lying

This is a completely thrilling inquiry. At the component even as you contact your face, the pores and pores and skin on your arms is sensitive to touch and becomes redder. This is referred to as the bloodstream and is multiplied whilst we lie.

The justification in the lower back of that is that the man or woman lying will experience remorseful and they'll start to perspire. Sweat creates a tingle that brings approximately humans contacting their faces to ease it.

It's important to take word that this signal is not 100% real as it very well may be applied as a way for trickiness with the beneficial aid of the folks that are first-rate at what they do like talented poker game enthusiasts, entertainers, and legislators.

Recall that we need to peruse agencies of statistics and that no person's non-verbal conversation hobby can show someone is deceptive us.

The Eyes

While it's miles tough to be aware absolutely at the off hazard that someone is mendacity, a few caution signs will give you a very top notch estimate.

Eye dispositions are probable the handiest technique for seeing, assuming any character is mendacity. Assuming eye dispositions toward the mouth or forehead increment when they communicate, this will display that they may be creating a splendid try to make their story doable.

Individuals who lie regularly gaze upward and to the right greater regularly than dad and mom which might be being sincere, which scientists assume may be due to the reality liars try and concoct what they'll say straightaway. More on eye development underneath and why it very well can be valid or bogus depending upon the individual.

Seeing Changes In The Eyes

It is not possible to apprehend if every person is lying with their eyes.

The maximum widely identified rationalization that people take delivery of is that liars will avoid the eye to eye connections. We disagree with that assertion. A liar will take care of your facts and hold a close to eye on you to test whether you have got become worried with the untruth. If a few issue, sanctuaries won't live faraway from the attention-to-eye connection thru manner of any stretch of the creativeness, it is no longer in that body of mind to do such.

All human beings push aside or supply down their appears while now not wishing to rise as an awful lot as an editorial. This mollifies numerous feelings, like misery, obligation, and loathing. Liars except can also want to offer little symptoms and signs and symptoms of evasion, seeing as they probable are conscious no man or woman hopes to have the choice to peer duplicity inside the eyes.

Pupil Dilation

Pupils dilate whilst human beings are sincerely excited, however there can be no willful pathway that lets in certainly every body the selection to go along with this alteration by using the use of preference.

Pupil dilation is created by manner of the autonomic sensory machine.

While expanded student dilation is often related with feeling inspired, it does no longer permit us to understand the individual inclination.

Crying

It's no longer surprising to cry while driven, but, crying might no longer generally mean an character is miserable. Tears stand up in snapshots of pain, bitterness, assist, or an entire lot of laughing.

On the off threat that any person is in fact crying, their eyebrows need to likewise flow into or provide signs of dampness, as well. You need to have the option to experience the dampness in the back of the tears, on the off hazard that you do no longer, this is a few exclusive statistics factor nicely worth exploring. Noticing.

Not all tears are legitimate.

Squint Rate Change

Is squinting a ton an illustration of lying? You can sample any character's flicker fee and be aware an increment at the same time as they're below strain. The widespread squint price is someplace within the fashion of 8 and twenty instances every second.

On the off chance that you see an growth in flicker rate, that is an area of electricity for a thing and one not to be excused.

The flickering reflex, which can not be stifled deliberately, is a crucial autonomic way of behaving that does not commonly order hobby. We can put it to use for our ability benefit whilst dissecting a few non-verbal conversation.

At the component whilst a squint rate transforms, we recognize a few thing has modified inner. We want to offer extra attention to this to look what's occurring.

Non-verbal conversation Lying Looking To The Right

Head traits are a large a part of appears, they're an lousy lot of the time oblivious dispositions which may be made with out a cognizant plan. We make head tendencies to offer our viewpoints or emotions approximately what we see or hear in the weather.

Assuming you spot the top skip to at least one thing or the eyes drop right down to the proper this will show a profound response to a few component stated or recommended.

It's essential to speak about the scenario beforehand of time and dive into the setting extraordinarily more.

Non-verbal verbal exchange Lying Looking To The Left

We've all visible humans on TV, in motion photos, or in our private lives who appear to return clean through their non-verbal conversation. They shake their head left and proper to mention "No" once they advise "Yes." In all reality any head improvement isn't confident to illustrate mendacity all on my own. On the off chance that you be conscious a change in behavior and it's far interior multiple moments of the initial time, this may imply trickery. Notwithstanding, you want to peruse non-verbal communication in corporations of information, so you can get a awesome translation of the circumstance.

Exemplary Body Language Signs Of Lying

There are severa exemplary caution signs of mendacity consist of: deflected eye-to-eye connection, elevated gulping, counterfeit grin, shallow respiratory, and shortage of appears.

Is Touching The Ear A Sign Of Lying

Individuals utilize this movement when they be given as true with they have been trapped in a fake or pursued a horrible preference and need to get away from it as fast as may be predicted. This is mentioned within the non-verbal conversation international as a pacifier or self-mitigating behavior. It is pretty vital whilst you word any person contacting their ear on the same time as being addressed.

Recollect that there are not any absolutes. We need to constantly peruse companies of facts and recognize one piece of non-verbal verbal exchange cannot display urgency all by myself.

Brain science Body Language Signs Of Lying

Understanding the human thoughts is not any easy undertaking. A few critical such things as what forms of meals are extremely good for you, what rest manner on your intellectual prosperity, and the manner to inform on the same time as you're in risk are a few vital facts that people need to be aware of.

The critical functionality of the cerebrum is to hold messages starting with one spot and then onto the following. The messages are despatched through a shape of electrical signal known as a neuron. Neurons ship messages and speak them from one area in the thoughts and ship them to some different.

Our minds make a compound circuit that continues changing and transferring every time we connect to people. Each time we strive to kind out the difficulty they will be trying to say, we furthermore supply to them those messages once more.

There is not any smooth approach for telling and assuming that someone is deceiving us. If there had been no humans, they would not make it seem.

Non-verbal communique experts unique that there are sure symptoms to recollect while you are trying to apprehend lies.

Above all else, recognize about their eye-to-eye connection. On the off hazard that they shy away or squint extra than predicted, they may be deceptive you. They can also furthermore likewise deflect their appearance more than expected, that is another sign that they are not coming clean.

Assuming they appear to be perspiring extra than expected or giving indicators of uneasiness like scouring their fingers collectively or squirming excessively, the ones may also want to likewise reveal that they'll be not being straightforward with you.

In end, assuming the man or woman feels awkward in a few manner or each different and is using more hand motions, for instance, this may advise that a few factor is off-base and it's miles the right opportunity a good way to discover similarly.

Chapter 4: Obstacles To Finding The Truth

The Barrier to Truth

I stand by way of using the usage of being attentive to the statistics, I stand through being attentive to the legislators, I track in (outwardly) to posts on Facebook and I truely can not recognize wherein to music down fact.

In fact, there's no reality. There is my truth, and your reality, and beginning these days once I checked, more than a 7.8billion human beings have insights throughout the globe. What we find within the international is in truth a discernment due to how our mind is careworn out - it's far a assembly - and every cerebrum in the world is harassed all of sudden.

To beat this, widely known what you pay interest from others as a planning stage, no longer an endpoint.

The unequalled boundary to the fact of the problem is proactive hobby. The shortfall of proactive interest leaves us defenseless in opposition to being 'indoctrinated' i.E., tolerating non-truth or supposition as fact. This is everyday for people, clearly now not specially precious. It is likewise a robust political tool - international governmental troubles in addition to fellowship circle governmental troubles.

The Biggest Obstacle to Truth:

Why Feelings Need to be Put Aside Before Entering Discussion

"He who realizes each one of the responses has now not been published every one of the inquiries" — Confucius

That's what the idiom goes on the off hazard which you do no longer want to have displeased visitors, then, at that factor, you need to in no manner talk legislative troubles or religion at an night accumulating. We can increase this rundown of no issues to troubles encompassing profound fine, as an example, early termination and killing simply to provide a few examples.

These elements supply with their convictions and views which can be regularly well set up and whenever tested, can also spark off the exhilaration of quite unmistakable tendencies. Such sentiments can be a demonstration of ethical fact and want to probable be a mark of profound apprehend.

Notwithstanding this, in spite of the fact that, it stays the continually gift fact that the ones properly-established sentiments are an obstacle to finding reality.

Before we're capable of make clear further why we need to jettison our sentiments taking component in moral discussions, we need to pose ourselves a simply applicable inquiry — What is profound best?

"We are speaking approximately no little rely, but the manner that we should live" — Socrates, In Plato's Republic

What is Morality?

Commonly referred to as the number one ethical scholar, Socrates as quickly as permit us to apprehend the issue of moral great arrangements with "No little rely amount, but how we have to stay."

Moral manner of thinking endeavors to distinguish proper from off-base, outstanding from awful, and moral from evil.

There isn't any all-inclusive, uncontroversial this means that of what ethical awesome is, with numerous books embracing rival hypotheses with reference to residing an moral existence. Amidst each this sort of contending definitions, Socrates' number one plan of profound incredible has the beneficial beneficial resource of no longer culpable or disproving considered certainly one of a type definitions set ahead and it's far the definition that we will push in advance with.

Ethical first-rate isn't always any little hold in mind, but how we must live.

Jettison your sentiments

Recollect the closing warmed verbal exchange you have been a bit of. Picture the very last time you enthusiastically protected a mind-set you regular to be the unassailable truth.

It may want to now not be too unreasonable on my issue to foresee that there may be a excellent opportunity you finished the communicate retaining exactly the identical evaluation which you entered the conversation with.

Certain components of our convictions are settled to such an extent that they uphold unimaginably overwhelming inclinations whilst examined and as in recent times discovered, those overwhelming inclinations can now and again display a specific moral earnestness that allows you to be dependable. By and via, however, unmistakable dispositions are often not beneficial for looking for reality — a preference that need to be a part of every one oldsters.

At the detail whilst we've got were given a enterprise opinion approximately an problem, it's far unimaginably appealing to count on that we genuinely apprehend what reality must be, without pondering the contentions introduced on the opportunity facet.

"He who realizes each one of the responses has not published every one of the inquiries." — Confucius

Yet, may additionally need to we at any point depend on the ones sentiments to provide us truth? It appears to be no longer.

Our sentiments may be off-base, regardless of how robust they is probably. Our sentiments is probably silly, they will brush aside hundreds of the motive that we've muddled to maintain our mind-set upstanding. They is probably risky, loaded up with heuristics and predispositions, and went down thru a long term of individuals in our organization of buddies.

Sentiments are an awful lot of the time the consequences of bias and social molding. The strain of social molding is regularly subverted. We need to not fail to recollect there has been a duration quite these days all through the whole lifestyles of mankind, where humans' 'sentiments' allow them to apprehend that it emerge as affordable to shop for and skip down character humans within the maximum over-the-pinnacle grievous and de-refining fashion. Indeed, even these days, the sensations of severa in the public vicinity permit them to realise that it's miles ethically first-rate to take conscious cognizant animals from their youngsters, deal with them inside the maximum probably woeful way, before finishing their attention, so we're able to have meat at some stage in supper. What will our own family say regarding this form of idea?

Simply take a gander at the stress of social molding on our 'sentiments' and ask your self again whether or not our sentiments may be depended upon always.

Use motivation to motive

Assuming seeking out the records of the hassle is our vital purpose, we should try and allow our sentiments to be directed through manner of the contentions we are able to provide for contradicting mind. We need to invite mind in opposition to our private with terrific affection as a treasured opportunity to draw one level toward reality.

Human bias is a place of energy so it often appears as a preference for non-threatening statistics. Frequently we need to simply accept a story because it upholds our previous attitude.

A communist will want to accept contentions that area employee's guilds in a remarkable moderate. An entrepreneur will need to agree with contentions for the de-guiding principle of the unrestricted financial system and confined authorities.

Yet, modern realities and reality-esteem exist freely of our dreams and dreams, and conscious moral reasoning can start as soon as we set our biases to the element.

"The sincere moral professional is a person who's worried pretty with the pursuits of surely all people impacted with the useful resource of what the man or woman does; who carefully filters realities and analyzes their hints; who recognizes necessities of lead completely after analyzing them to make certain they'll be sound: who will "yield to not unusual feel" in any occasion, even as it approach that in advance convictions would possibly need to be reexamined; and who, at final, will follow up on the outcomes of this interest"

— Dr. James Rachels, The Elements of Moral Philosophy

Chapter 5: How To Investigate The Truth

7 Ways to Get on the Truth in a Workplace Investigation

Joined with education and experience, the proper gadgets would possibly probable become being the professionals crucial to the vault

#1 Read the Suspect's Behavior

A superb questioner searches for verbal and non-verbal suggestions. "You will stand with the resource of paying attention to what they say in addition to how they will be announcing it, how they are sitting, how they may be responding with their frame language, Everybody's modified into a representative within the non-verbal communique techniques because of TV. On the off threat which you peer down and to the left you have to lie. In any case, that is faux all of the time.

It's a social event of this statistics at the same time as you're sitting contrary someone."

Although there aren't any simple responses, honest suspects are via and massive more direct, Most guiltless people will reply indignantly to go-to-head a showdown. "They will say you are insane, I had now not something to do with it." Guilty people will greater regularly than not be more uninvolved throughout the bypass-exam, he says.

#2 Use Positive Confrontation

Among the strategies for uplifting an admission, a amazing showdown is commonly utilized with a suspect you are taking transport of is blameworthy.

"Positive showdown is largely what it recommends: that you are persuaded of the man or woman's obligation and you could face them with it. You will look for a suspect's way of behaving. Could it be said that they're feeble? Do they supply unconvincing refusals?"

#3 Cast Blame Away from the Suspect

Projecting fault on a person else or state of affairs might in all likelihood draw you closer to an admission. "You can provide them an partner: 'Clearly you did not do this with the useful aid of itself. You can fault joblessness for making the individual want the cash. Or then again, fault their unlucky reimbursement. You can endorse the corporation brings in all of the coins on earth and they will be capable of go through the fee of it,

"What you're truely attempting to find is some thing they may reply to."

#four Establish Control

"During bypass-examination, the questioner have to lay out manipulate of the talk. You need to count on disavowals at some stage in the meeting or move-examination,

Try no longer to permit interferences. "Their mouth might be open like they want to mention some factor… they may repair the eye to eye connection,or boost their hand while you are speaking like they need to almost increase their hand to talk," he says.

#5 Use Objections as Opportunities

Numerous protests, whenever taken in a real experience, are honest. A difficulty would in all likelihood say "I like my career plenty to do that" or "I might be excessively worrying to conform with through with a few aspect like that."

"It's the open door you're looking for because of the fact you could then say: 'I'm happy you said that. I receive as real with that is legitimate, You can likewise have a look at up and express something such that 'this we could me realise this isn't something you made arrangements for pretty a while. This is clearly a few issue that happened, and that is the cause it's so vital to get this defined due to the reality you cope with it like your business enterprise,"

#6 Keep the Subject's Attention

There are many stunts to preserve the difficulty's hobby, contingent upon wherein you are within the bypass-examination. "

If they have got given a portion of the signs of regret or contemptibility you can slide your seat closer, Sometimes - seldom and most probable supplied that there is someone else inside the room and its similar sex - you may contact the person on the arm and deal some solace. What's more, you want to try and restore the eye to eye connection on the off risk that they may be peering down."

#7 Ask Alternative Questions

A couple of tough questions can get you to admission all the greater proficiently. For example: Did you take 20,000 or 30,000 or was it an lousy lot less?

"By and big it's miles clever to misrepresent due to the truth many people will hop on that and say 'no I just took 500 dollars. It sounds mindless but it appears after enterprise." You need to result in the suspect to extensively recognized one of the higher options you are giving, he says.

Introducing information such that the suspect can admit with best a number one gesture of the pinnacle is possible too. For instance: "So you in all likelihood did not take 30,000 dollars you took 500 greenbacks, is that right?"

There are numerous strategies of checking the honesty of a meeting trouble, but, there are dependably particular instances, Someone also can have a terrible day. Somebody can also have recently misplaced a pal or member of the family. Furthermore, in an effort to affect this huge tremendous style of tells."

Indeed, regardless of every one of the suggestions and deceives reachable, there's no reliable method for purchasing human beings to return back returned smooth with you. In any case, joined with guidance and experience, the proper apparatuses also can become being the examiner's vital to the vault. The reliably carried out exam approach is critical to making fantastic a covered running surroundings weather, however, what happens even as you suspect any character isn't always coming easy at some stage in an examination? Harvard Business Review research suggests that we as an entire lie from time to time, and the ordinary individual lies instances in step with day. Nonetheless, it's far one factor to guarantee that you skipped dessert or completed your interest assembly (at the same time as you probably did not) — it's far some aspect else in reality while your misleading case might also moreover have an effect on the place of business round you and your pals.

Questioners ought to try to guarantee that openness is a want of any speak during the investigatory cycle. Somebody's art work and vocation would possibly depend upon how topics become, so all members need to stick with genuineness. At the problem at the same time as there are signs and symptoms and symptoms that a worker isn't always coming smooth, the accompanying advances guide managers in the method closer to an OK cease quit result.

Plan Questions Carefully

Stage one: Start each meeting via auditing assumptions approximately the requirement for trustworthiness while responding to questions and the ramifications for now not doing as such. Making this the start level of the interaction for all representative meetings, units the policies further to communicates some issue precise that everyone is being held to a similar norm.

The approach of the examiner isn't always to investigate observers and people — this isn't a courtroom. All subjects being identical, the eye need to be on posing all-around created questions to determine whether or no longer solutions are sincere or not. Trustworthy responses result in better examination outcomes, while misleading statements and precise misrepresentations, if no longer wonderful, can swiftly screw up any headway you are making towards a reason.

Part of the way to improvement is being key about the inquiries you pose. Inquiring "positive" or "no" questions does now not permit you to accumulate appropriate subtleties. Begin substantially and in a while tight toward the number one detail in need of interest. On the off hazard that you begin with "the vital issue" without skipping a beat, you are positive to have the worker solution out of dread or apprehension. Warm up with harmless inquiries regarding paintings connections and special first rate focuses earlier than hopping into the greater profound quantities of the discussion.

Inspect and Verify the Facts

Asking look at-up inquiries or rewording your inquiries assists with ensuring a truely specific response. This is useful for documentation functions but moreover assists with ensuring the employee simply comprehends the difficulty and isn't converting the tale midway.

If you get clashing information, it's miles viable the interviewee is being untruthful. For example, if key realities alternate in addition to complex memories are applied to hide a alternate inside the tale, those are warnings for distortion. Test rather greater profoundly with follow-up inquiries to ensure you have got an unmistakable photo and regular (or conflicting) subtleties. If everything which you are saying simply does not make any enjoy, do no longer rise as an awful lot because the interviewee, but alternatively confirm the story within its maximum cutting-edge emphasis. Your subsequent degree is to survey the interviewee's story closer to first rate handy proof. For example, assuming that there are messages, information, witness articulations, or one in every of a type kinds of statistics to affirm or go towards the record, those bits of proof might be large to the examination effects.

Follow the Process

If you stumble into someone that in all likelihood won't be coming easy, they must no longer get an exchange method or approach than the the relaxation of the contributors.

For every meeting, the intention is to build up information and illustrate what came about. Assuming any individual is being untruthful and it turns into exposed, there may be a appropriate chance to control that.

On the off hazard which you suspect deceptive proclamations had been made, lead a subsequent meeting. The object is to all in all examine the interviewee's specific announcement and proposition and open doorways for clarifications of the irregularities in mild of recent proof or records you may have located. Your manner is to decide whether the clashing statement have grow to be the interviewee mendacity or the end result of some one-of-a-type clarification like a difference in discernment or perhaps a mitigating scenario. For example, you could take a look at that a totally unique misleading declaration became made because of a worry about reprisal.

Go with a Choice and Take Action

How would not it no longer be an fantastic concept an exquisite way to reply on the off hazard which you verify the consultant is being unscrupulous? After the exam is completed, direct your interest in the direction of handling the principle scenario. Very much like any presentation trouble, the discussions you have got got and the sports activities sports you're taking should be exhaustively stated.

The following level is to think about turning into disciplinary interest. While it'd seem like attainable to take an outrageous response, be fine the place suits the situations. Contingent on the degree of the double-dealing, the prevent might be the proper sport-plan. Nonetheless, there can be conditions at the same time as a composed censure, or maybe a quick suspension to build up the concept that untrustworthiness isn't some factor to be messed with, is more appropriate. These requirements are to rise up ultimately later and want to be truely recorded to avoid any appearance of indecency or reprisal.

Chapter 6: Examining Right Or Wrong People

How Can I Know Right From Wrong?

Before we are able to apprehend the way to advantage ethical know-how, we need to first recognise the individual of the requirements that are being stated on every occasion we speak what constitutes precise and evil. A non-naturalist rationalization of morality, to begin with placed forth by way of way of G.E. Moore in his Principia Ethica, is the type of account that I want to offer proper right here (1903). In the manner of lifestyles of Moore, we would think about morality as having a shape of often taking place measurement. Every motion may be placed somewhere along this moral measurement, which degrees from the maximum one of a type characteristic to the most vice, with a medium floor of neutrality in among.

Permit me to now examine morality to the passage of time. There isn't always any tangible feature of the arena that we're capable of element to that demonstrates the passage of time itself. On the alternative hand, we do now not need on the manner to element to some thing concrete as a manner to understand that factor passes. Instead, it is the truth that our highbrow capacities had been advanced particularly to sense the passage of time that gives the affect that point has a extra impact on us. This appears to be real with regard to morals as well. We aren't pointing to a bodily entity of "wrongness" at the equal time as we witness a murder and say that it is wrong; rather, we are highlighting a cost this is inherent inside the witnessed motion. For instance, at the same time as we witness a murder and say that it is wrong, we're pointing to the truth that the murder is wrong. The moral difficulty leaves an impact on us in the form of way that allows us to recognize the tendencies of morality.

If we're capable of apprehend moral truths in this way, then one should question how there can no matter the truth that be plenty controversy around ethical problems. But no longer all factors of morality may be summed up as succinctly as "killing is incorrect" and "being useful is right." One might argue that because someone might also moreover have the right to homicide some other person on the manner to prevent the explosion of a bomb in a university, one might argue that killing isn't always continuously morally incorrect. There are many high-quality motives and portions of records that lie inside the heritage that contribute to moves. We want to realise now not just the motion itself however moreover the purpose, the thoughts-set of the person carrying out the motion, and the quit result that that they'd in mind when they carried it out if you want to decide whether or not or now not a few problem complicated is moral. The moral knowledge of someone can be determined via the use of manner of gauging the reactions they need to an movement, similarly to via studying the notion strategies of the person who performed the deed. Some people are extra adept at taking in these sensations and then remodeling them into know-how than others. This is not to raise ethicists to the location of moral priesthood, but. My lecturer in metaethics in evaluation it to region, explaining that someone who is spatially unaware can also run the threat of bumping their heads on matters often. Learning a manner to nicely interpret our moral perceptions is one of the outstanding methods for any oldsters to improve our expertise of morality.

Manly, Auckland, New Zealand resident Julian Shields

There isn't always any foolproof approach, however there may be a path that can be located that can be of assist in precarious instances. First matters first, get all the facts approximately the scenario. Lack of knowledge in no manner ends in clever choice-making. Allow specific humans to tell you of factors that you would possibly choose to neglect about. Try to assume the results of any sports activities you can take, that is a much greater hard step than the first. Unfortunately, even precisely expected consequences may want to possibly have unintentional knock-on outcomes that have been now not expected. However, even the most ardent proponent of non-consequentialism is needed to do not forget the effects of their actions because supporting unique people is a crucial moral fantastic, regardless of the reality that it is not the maximum important one. Examine the ethical precepts that direct you to behave in a tremendous manner or every different, due to the fact the 1/3 step on this approach. These standards need to be accurate at the identical time as additionally being applicable, which is some component that might be debated. The Catholic Church holds the view that divorce is morally incorrect, however Islamic regulation makes it smooth for men to divorce their better halves. You take delivery of as actual with that we must understand the sanctity of without a doubt all and sundry's lifestyles, even the life of a assassin, however I agree with that murderers have abandoned the concept of the sanctity of life. Take the plunge and make the choice.

Unfortunately, actual and relevant moral requirements struggle, and we can also moreover should pick amongst assertions which may be similarly vital so that you can determine which one we ought to adhere to. Taking a utilitarian attitude, I undergo in mind that the goal that contributes the most quantity of particular to the world want to be taken into consideration the maximum great one. However, this is not commonly the case. I actually have a larger duty to positive humans than to others, which conflicts with the obligation I must shop as many lives as feasible in choice to fewer. Yet, I will pick to hold my non-public teenager over 10 everyday strangers. The concept of morality sprang from the idea of kinship, and we want no longer wander too an extended manner from its origins. There is likewise the possibility that great concepts are inherently extra vast than others. It's feasible that it is more critical not to take a existence than it's miles to store one, in which case I need to refuse to take the lifestyles of 1 man or woman as a manner to save . But what if I simply want to sacrifice one life to keep fifty? There is not this type of issue as absolute morality; rather, morality may be applicable to at least one's sports, and in the long run, the utilitarian principle prevails. It is useful to do an assessment of parallel situations wherein the solution is obvious; analyzing how these conditions variety from the issue available simplifies questioning. And do not forget to address problems both with people whose evaluations you recognize and with individuals who are in competition in your very personal. If you're making a mistake, you need to forgive your self and artwork on being better the following time.

Allen Shaw, Harewood, Leeds

Because conformity to a middle moral precept so regularly seems to provide a solid foundation upon which to assemble ethical conduct, one of the most effective methods to reply to this trouble can be to take a look at extensively held ethical beliefs and be aware how properly they comply with to the situation to be had. The Golden Rule, often called' do unto others as you'll have them do unto you, 'is an instance of the kind of necessities. This idea may be placed in masses of precise religions and belief systems. The argument that mind like this one might also feature correct publications to determining what constitutes "proper" and "wrong" is compelling. Some moralists maintain the notion that a feel of duty, in location of a herbal propensity to behave ethically, is the deliver of moral behavior. It does appear to be ethically useful to renowned one's obligations to others in place of one's very very very own self-interest. In addition, thinkers who're caused through Kant argue that we ought to now not see distinctive people as "certainly a technique to a aim," however as an alternative as "ends in themselves," admitting that other people are capable of ethical mirrored image. It may want to appear that treating humans as absolutely a purpose in desire to a technique is the morally accurate factor to do because it demonstrates altruism and respect for first rate human beings, each of which are probable fairly full-size attributes in accurate moral behavior.

Nevertheless, the stringent software program program of moral norms might in all likelihood result in effects that appear immoral. The massive majority of people feel that lying is usually terrible however that there are fantastic instances in which it's miles perfect to reap this, which encompass at the same time as searching for to store someone's existence. Second, putting an emphasis at the importance of duty can supply the influence that ethics is hard and counter-intuitive, which isn't always without a doubt convincing; it appears hard to criticize a obviously generous man or woman for now not being clearly moral due to the reality they do no longer act out of a experience of duty. This is due to the fact it's miles counter-intuitive to don't forget that ethics is traumatic and requires going in the direction of one's natural instincts. In surrender, however the fact that the exquisite majority of human beings may need to agree that we ought to admire and cherish the human beings round us, we is probably willing to tolerate treating other humans as a technique if the result is probable to have plenty greater excellent consequences. For example, an entire lot of humans think it's miles okay to kill one man or woman with a view to keep a set of diverse human beings's lives and that it's miles in truth lousy not to perform that if you could assist it. It may also seem that humans, regardless of the reality that they frequently have amazing feelings that illustrate to them even as a specific movement is appropriate or beside the point, moreover famend that there are times wherein a rigid adherence to the equal standards can be complicated and/or unethical. This suggests that ethics is simply as uncertain as any other subfield of philosophy. Because of this, making definitive moral judgments about what is right and incorrect can be tough, and as a result, many ethical troubles are although open.

Jonathan Tipton of Preston, Lancashire

Philosophers might likely argue approximately a great sort of thoughts, however in the end, I do not forget that a honest boo-hurrah approach is the brilliant manner to decide what is right and what is incorrect. Okay, i'll admit that I'm no longer taking psychopaths into attention. Nevertheless, I should contend that the large majority of people on earth are born with an constructed in ethical code that reasons them to cringe in revulsion from immoral conduct. This code is rooted in empathy. Simply ask yourself if that is the way you would love to be handled so that you can decide whether or not or not or now not your movements in the direction of every other individual are appropriate or inappropriate.The objectivity lies inside the fact that we are dwelling, aware animals. Why make subjects any greater complex than that?

Urmston, Manchester, and Morgan Millard had been noted.

It is feasible to attract the belief from the question that the capacity to distinguish amongst tremendous and wrong is largely cognitive. Consequently, the usage of the language of Benjamin Bloom's taxonomy of educational dreams in the cognitive region, I am capable of take into account topics that have been declared suitable or beside the point, and I am capable of recognize the reasons why they're appropriate or beside the point. I can follow my recollection and comprehension of right and wrong to behave efficiently in precise events; I can analyze behaviors and decide which is probably right and incorrect; I can examine why a few are right or incorrect; and I can create more finely nuanced conceptions of rightness or wrongness.This information have turn out to be acquired via the system of trial and errors further to by using inferring it from the responses of different people to the things that I do or say.

However, it is also a rely of emotion because of the truth the responses of various humans to what I say or do motive feelings to upward push up internal me. To practice Bloom's idea to this area, I first be aware about or make a intellectual word of pleasant behaviors that elicit reactions from one of a kind people or feelings in myself. I get the functionality to react as it should be in great conditions when others do positive movements. Additionally, I get the effect that fantastic remarks are favored more distinctly through specific human beings than on my own. Some of those rather desired replies are prepared via me consistent with a set of ideas. In the give up, the ones guiding thoughts are interdependent, and as a quit give up result, my conduct is defined through them.

For instance, at the same time as my mom first of all positioned me at her breast, I did so out of a natural inclination to satiate my starvation. On the opportunity hand, I skilled the fun of satiety, of warmth, and of safety. I sobbed each time I became thirsty or chilly, after which if I was scared. I determined out that this woman have to meet those requirements whenever they arose. Then, through coincidence, my toothless jaws performed too much strain to the nipple. My mom, startled, took a step all over again, and withdrew the meals from the desk. I shed some tears, after which the deliver turn out to be restored. I paid interest to those topics, and I recalled the following: I spoke back to maternal acts; I took word that in reaction to positive of my moves, she need to deliver gadgets that delivered satisfaction, but in reaction to exceptional actions, her response supplied heaps a whole lot much less pleasure. I received an information of the subjects that have been essential to my mother and the assets of her satisfaction for me. In this way, she modified into organising what emerge as superb and incorrect. As my language skills improved, I started out out to conceptualize the ones mind and, thru communication together collectively with her and, in the end, with increasingly other humans, I polished those conceptions. The social interactions that take region among different people and me establish what constitutes proper and incorrect. They want to advantage expertise of. Because I favored to suit in with society, I had to educate myself and adopt its requirements of what constitutes well and awful behavior.

Alasdair Macdonald, Glasgow

As an character, I am born right into a society that calls for obedience to a set of legal guidelines and norms by means of way of which I did now not select to be positive. This is the case no matter the truth that I did now not want to be part of this society. In order to coexist peacefully with my fellow residents, it's far required of me to conduct myself in a positive way and to stick to a hard and fast of norms. Assuming I do now not have any form of intellectual disease, I have to start to gather those social standards at a greater youthful age via my affiliations with corporations, which can in the end bring about the formation of my cultural identity. In my roles as a member of a family, a church, a kingdom, an educational agency, and an occupational putting, I am knowledgeable in the customs, values, and suggestions of these affiliations. For example, as a extra younger family member, I take a look at via the route of my parents that it is beside the point to act spitefully within the direction of siblings and that modeling appropriate conduct is a brilliant manner to set a excellent example for more youthful siblings, who may additionally observe the distinction among right and incorrect from me. Because I am an adult, I am required to signal an employment contract, and if I do now not, I hazard losing my hobby. As a self-enough person, I obtain responsibility for my sports, collectively with the corporation I preserve and the people I accomplice with. I can also moreover begin to question my determined out behaviors and morals after being uncovered to other cultures, moralities, and notion structures. I also can cause as to whether or not or now not I desire to hold those institutions, weighing the results of discontinuing what I understand and attaching myself to new institutions and organizations, consisting of changing my faith and the effect that this can have on my own family and buddies. For instance, I also can start to question whether or not or no longer or not I choice to keep those associations. However, in trendy, I am able to distinguish among fantastic and incorrect because of the identification connections I definitely have advanced at some point of my lifestyles. This lets in me to simply accept duty for the consequences of the selections I make as an character. There is a capability for friction: as an instance, positive societies condone the exercise of "honor murders," whilst others insist that it's miles by no means perfect to take each different person's life. What ought to you do if, no matter the reality that the rules of the network in which you stay forbid honor murders, you are a part of a way of life that encourages the exercise of such killings? If you're making the aware selection to

111

interrupt together together with your preceding affiliations, you may want to face jail effects.

Sharon Painter is a Rugeley, Staffordshire resident.

Simply positioned, I am unable to. Not in any manner that can be actually tested. The thoughts of accurate and wrong are creations, the effects of an evolving sense of self-consciousness. This is in assessment to the policies of physics, which keep to carry out no matter whether or now not or not or now not humans realise them. Nietzsche continues that our capability for rational idea has advanced an extended way later than our primal tendencies. Examining attitudes closer to killing is a superb way to demonstrate the ramifications of this locating. The concept of "murder" as a criminal offense might probable were incomprehensible to early people. Because it become essential to kill so as to live alive, "murder" have come to be an familiar and herbal a part of normal life. The only detail that diminished the urge to kill in self-safety modified into the transition from hunter-gatherer lives to installed societies. This marked the start of the regular march toward the popularity that murder is unethical. However, there may be a seize on this sentence. Many humans are of the opinion that there are instances even as killing is appropriate. Even in conditions that appear to have a easy solution, it's miles difficult to inform for splendid what is right and what is inaccurate because of the life of such ambiguities. However, the equal precept applies in specific contexts. In spite of the reality that I recollect many acts to be repugnant and morally repugnant, it is viable to discover times in which they were traditionally suitable. At a few thing in human statistics, humans have stopped questioning rape, thievery, and one in every of a type forms of persecution.

It is handiest possible to bypass judgement in retrospect because of the reality that suitable and wrong do not exist independently of the collective awareness of the human beings of the planet at a particular instantaneous. We may argue that moving perspectives are proof of an inherent 'wrongness' especially movements, probable pointing to a natural order of proper and wrong in a way that is similar to the discovery of prison tips of physics. But comparable ideals had been showed to be incorrect inside the past. It was believed for millennia that religious texts furnished definitive solutions. However, if a writer had been to show themselves and say such things as "Same-sex marriage is inaccurate" or "Capital punishment is right," many human beings, which include myself, could have a very tough time accepting those statements. We all at once had a organisation keep near on what have come to be proper and incorrect, but we had the impact that many stuff taken into consideration "right" were absolutely "incorrect," and vice versa.

Although there are perhaps effective elements of accurate and evil which is probably obvious, the majority of the time, it's far as an awful lot as us to conform with our enjoy of right and incorrect. Because of this, not some aspect may be said for unique. Simply stated, I want to supply it my all.

Located in Sutton in Ashfield, Nottinghamshire is Glenn Bradford.

To solution your query in a nutshell, no, I can't. According to Dr. Oliver Scott Curry of Oxford University, he has, in essence, solved the problem of morality thru reading empirical facts from sixty one-of-a-type civilizations, each historic and present day-day. My interpretation of his first mind is provided inside the following, which means that that he ought to get the random e-book.

In the identical way that Rome became built on seven hills, morality is based totally mostly on seven values that have organically evolved through time and are held to severa levels. The purposes of these values are to each sell collaboration or solve warfare. The maximum crucial of those is ownership, which 9 out of ten awesome cultures and the prison tool keep to be sacred. Following that, kinship, loyalty, and reciprocity are ideas which might be supported with the useful useful resource of three-quarters of the respondents. Respect (for the effective) and humility are fairly valued in more than 1/2 of the sector's civilizations (of the powerless). Fairness is to be had in lifeless last, accounting for most effective 15% of the entire fee.Therefore, socialism have to be prevented, and one need to in no manner offer a idiot a straightforward hazard. The crux of the problem is that there are not any opportunity ethical requirements. Each person has their private unique set of guiding necessities, similarly to their very very own aesthetic judgment, but there are best seven middle values that may surely be shared.

The seven tenets of morality are interpreted in lots of contexts and given severa ranges of significance with the aid of numerous countries and cultures. What is proper is what contributes to the accomplishment of some purpose, whether or not that aim be replica, social cohesiveness, a long lifestyles, affluence, or victory. Wrong is what gets within the manner of carrying out the goal, and committing evil is visible as purposefully being in the way. It's viable that specific people's values are in conflict with each different, which can also bring about disturbing recollections. What if the aim is to workout typical dominance over entire surrender for the relaxation of eternity?

Little Sandhurst's very very non-public Dr. Nicholas B. Taylor

What are some responses that we may additionally provide to this question? First, we need to have already got a famous idea of what it's far to be "proper" and "wrong"; in any other case, we can not even start to solution this query. If we didn't, the query could not make any experience to us at all. But at the same time, we do not proportion the views of others on what constitutes "appropriate" and "wrong." If we recognize what is proper and wrong for ourselves, then sincerely all this is required human beings is to offer an reason behind what the ones phrases talk with at the equal time as we use them, after which others is probably able to supply an reason behind what they're regarding, and our seeming dispute might be resolved.

Despite this, we are not able to continue. We can also all have a have a look at an movement, be in complete agreement at the statistics, about what the motion consists of, and about the results it has, and however but fluctuate over whether or not or no longer or not the motion is accurate. This is because the information are aim. If that is the case, then there is no need in persevering with this argument concerning the individual of the movement that became taken. The deliver of our dispute – and, therefore, what we both understand to be "correct" – want to be a few other area. This permits supply an reason behind why we occasionally can not come to an agreement concerning the appropriateness of an hobby: the degree to which an motion is suitable can fine be appraised in comparison to brilliant acts. Which steps must we take then? If we were able to pick out the wonderful that set "right" sports aside from the others, we'd have additionally been able to outline what we meant whilst we spoke approximately right and incorrect behavior. But if that had been possible, then we might be once more to speakme approximately proper and incorrect close to some truth, and any seeming disagreements might be mounted to be not a few aspect greater than clean misunderstandings. But yet again, the reality that we're now not capable of reap a consensus indicates that this could no longer be the case. If correct and wrong are surely one among a type stages of the same system, and if we're unable to outline the boundaries of that device, then it follows that the device in question want to include the whole lot. What styles of systems try to encompass the entirety, or at least do their first-rate to perform that? Those relating philosophy: In light of this, I contend that our precise conceptions of what constitutes right and evil are long-established via the philosophies that we be a part of. If we're in possession of such an overarching philosophy, then we're already aware about what constitutes applicable and evil. If we do not have a employer keep close to on them, it is due to the fact our philosophical stances are not but completely evolved internal our personal thoughts.

John White, living in London.

Why ought to we assume that we're able to have the capacity to differentiate among proper and incorrect? It is a query of human desire, and particular human beings select to react to moral stressful situations in a whole lot of superb strategies. Morality isn't always hardwired into the cosmos in the identical manner that the legal guidelines of nature appear to be. Systems like Bentham's utilitarianism and Kant's deontology have essential insights, however they every have drawbacks as properly. The first has drawbacks because of its willful dismiss of the (assumed) rights of innocent human beings, and the second one has drawbacks due to its dismiss of the consequences of movements. But what exactly are we the use of as a diploma to evaluate the seeming shortcomings of those extremely good structures? Positivists trust that the difficulty is one in each of psychology and that it's miles encouraged via way of each

121

evolution and nurture. Does this ultimately result in relativism, with its inherent seeming contradiction that we need to never intrude within the affairs of a few distinctive manner of life or criticize a psychopath? It doesn't appear in all likelihood to me. The concept of subjecting innocent humans to useless suffering is repugnant within the majority of political systems. We are aware (or need to I say, maintain in thoughts?) That such harsh behavior is unacceptable because of some innate intellectual or emotional choice. And we are conscious that if we abide by means of the use of the use of sure necessities, our society will provide us with results which can be, to a extra or lesser extent, congruent with the ethical alternatives that we preserve. In many nations, a full-size a part of the population holds those beliefs, which helps foster a feel of shared task in the pursuit of morality. Why should not we try to influence special humans that the way of life that we have decided on is one that includes human intellectual interests, every theirs and ours?

This unified series of shared impulses, however, falls apart even as managing greater difficult conditions, along with abortion or one in all a type iterations of Phillipa Foot's "trolley conundrum." For those, there can be no consensus on what need to be completed, and we do now not have a tool for identifying, in a methodical or algorithmic manner, what the ideal response need to be. Any answer will skip closer to the internal intuition of at least one individual, and there may be no distinct way to measure how properly a desire-making machine works. We spend a whole lot of time annoying about the ones hard problems. It's viable that the question that needs to be requested isn't, "Did we find a answer that is ethically accurate?" while you don't forget that there may not be one, but as an alternative, "Did we fear over this trouble enough?" Have we wrangled with the problem and made positive that we've got looked at it from every attitude possible?

Is there a single, overarching criterion that can be used to differentiate among right and horrific? Doing the right problem is an act that adheres to morality, regulation, and justice, even as doing the wrong trouble is an act that doesn't adhere to morality or justice. In desired, doing the incorrect aspect refers to an act that breaks the law.

A correct motion is one that is legitimate, suitable, and proper, at the same time as an beside the point movement is one this is neither valid nor suitable. The proper movement is one that is legitimate and appropriate.

Some people maintain the view that moral thoughts and the functionality to make properly-considered picks aren't great, due to this that that they range depending on the tradition in question, and that there may be no one familiar ethical famous or capacity this is typically stated.

However, in preference to claiming that the thoughts' very natures are one-of-a-type, it may be extra accurate to statement that there are variations in the strategies wherein they'll be completed rather than to say that the ideas themselves are wonderful.

In antique Chinese manner of existence, kid's obligations closer to their parents intended one difficulty; in modern-day Western society, such duties suggest a few thing pretty special.

Nevertheless, appreciate for one's family and a spirit of cooperation are valued in every of these civilizations, further to nearly all others which is probably composed of human beings. In addition, there are various constraints positioned on individuals of a set or society from being able to do harm to amazing individuals of that organization or society in each way of life.

Every time we are in a feature in which we want to make a desire, we're properly conscious that there is a better and a worse opportunity to be had to us. Some alternatives have an effect on handiest the individual making them, including whether or no longer or no longer to position honey of their tea, even as others, such as being dishonest or stealing, have repercussions for unique human beings.

Therefore, how are we able to determine or justify which alternatives or behaviors are appropriate and which of them are beside the factor, in addition to which ones we can also or cannot perform?

There is a immoderate possibility that we might also all come to the realization that proper and wrong do no longer depend on a specific cause that is function of an movement or choice that determines whether or now not or no longer it is right or incorrect, nor that it's miles exceptional described with the aid of manner of conventions, civilizations, or the passage of time.

Of route, humans's traditions have the potential to direct and have an impact on their perceptions of what is ethically ideal or right. This is distinct from the argument that customs objectively decide what's proper or proper, because of the truth it is probably that positive behaviors and picks will preserve to live proper or wrong, despite the fact that the majority of the human beings worried do no longer acquire as genuine with them and accept as proper with they need to be adapted to cutting-edge times.

It is feasible that the incredible technique to reply to this hassle is to take the moral conceptions that are normally diagnosed and workout them to a specific situation in accordance with a huge moral precept that regularly serves as a honest basis for righteous conduct. One such idea is the Golden Rule of Confucius, which states, "Do unto others as you can have them do unto you," and is incorporated into a whole lot of unique belief structures and non secular traditions.

As an possibility to the perception that people are born with a herbal propensity to act morally, there are a few moralists who preserve the view that moral behavior derives from a sense of duty.

However, placing a strong emphasis at the importance of responsibility may moreover offer you with the affect that ethics is counter-intuitive, which isn't very convincing. It is probably tough to accuse a person who's truly giving of not being ethically sound due to the truth he or she does not act out of a feel of obligation. This is because of the reality someone who is obviously giving does now not act out of a feel of duty.

There isn't always all people method that might help people in distinguishing amongst right and incorrect, however there are numerous guidelines that may be useful in identifying the right route of motion while uncertainty arises.

The majority of people will first remember the capability consequences of their moves, and best then will they have got a examine the moral thoughts that may be gleaned from belongings that they keep in mind to be honest and pertinent. These assets can encompass customs, religion, culture, the legal machine, or something else that people recall to be massive and relevant.

Chapter 7: What Persuade People To Lie
The Reasons Behind the Telling of Lies

1. To stay out of trouble with the law. This is the justification that comes up most customarily even as humans speak approximately mendacity (by means of manner of each kids and adults). It is critical to word that there were no good sized versions among telling a lie to escape punishment for an intentional misdeed in vicinity of telling a deceive cowl up an sincere mistake close to the outcomes of the look at.

2. To advantage a prize that isn't with out problems obtained in every other way.Both youngsters and adults cite this as the second one maximum installation cause for their conduct. One example of this may be making up paintings revel in in the course of an interview for the cause of growing one's opportunities of getting the hobby.

Three. To guard every one of a kind character from the results in their actionsin the identical way that mendacity to keep away from private punishment does no longer modify motivation, proceeding does not have an impact on motive. This has occurred no longer without a doubt among employees but moreover with buddies, own family, and even whole strangers!

4. As a way to guard oneself from the opportunity of bodily harmthis is high-quality from being punished for the purpose that hazard of damage isn't in reaction to a wrongdoing at the a part of the character. One example of this would be a hint boy who is domestic by myself responding to a tourist on the door via announcing that his father is now dozing and they ought to pass returned later.

Five. In order to benefit the admiration of othersit is viable to tell "small white lies" to complement a tale that is being knowledgeable, or it is feasible to create a completely new (created) character even as you are mendacity to raise your recognition.

6. To free oneself from a difficult social situationexamples of the way telling falsehoods would possibly appear at the same time as they will be induced through using this encompass stating that you have issue locating a babysitter so you can break out from an uneventful birthday celebration, or stopping a cellular phone name through saying that there can be a person at the door. Both of these examples are lies.

7. To keep away from embarrassmentthe teenager who asserts that the moist seat have emerge as on account of water spilling and not because she wet her pants is an example of a little one who did now not fear being punished however instead felt embarrassed thru her conduct.

Eight. To shield one's anonymity with out informing some other birthday celebration of one's motive to gain this. For example, there is the couple that proclaims they eloped due to the fact the charge of a wedding changed into past their financial technique, however the reality is that they preferred to interrupt out the responsibility of inviting their circle of relatives to the rite.

Nine. To exert have an effect on on different humans via figuring out what records they've get right of get right of entry to to to and how they use it. This is probably the most perilous motive to tell a lie, and Hitler is a famous example of ways it can play out.

Still, more concept

I really have a sneaking suspicion that there are reasons for telling lies that don't wholesome into any of the nine education indexed above. These motives can also moreover additionally encompass petty deceits like falsehoods performed out of politeness or tact, which are not actually described via the aforementioned nine reasons. On the opportunity hand, those 9 were supplied in information that I for my part accumulated and might as a minimum function the idea for an proof of why people lie.

Keeping Oneself Out of Trouble

The motorist, who've turn out to be travelling 70 miles in keeping with hour, said to the police that he believed he have turn out to be only going fifty five miles in step with hour. "My wristwatch stopped, so I had no perception that I had come domestic hours after my curfew," the adolescent explains. "I had no concept that I had damaged my curfew." No recall what age they may be, humans of all ages perpetrate primary falsehoods for the most not unusual motive, it really is to avoid being punished in a few manner, whether or not or no longer or now not it is to avoid getting a dashing fee tag or being grounded. When one tells a excessive lie, they positioned themselves in chance of suffering huge damage if their deception is exposed. This may moreover furthermore embody the shortage of their freedom, coins, artwork, courting, reputation, or possibly existence.

Only in the most excessive of lies—the ones for which the liar should face punishment if caught—can mendacity be detected through mind-set, which incorporates facial capabilities, bodily movements, gaze, voice, or terms.The risk places an emotional burden on the reason, which might also additionally result in involuntary adjustments that would display the deception. The falsehoods of regular existence, wherein it would not remember number whether or not they'll be caught because of the fact there aren't any consequences or benefits, are an appropriate lies to tell without developing a unmarried mistake.

Keeping a Reward or Benefit Secret

When telling a big lie, the liar may frequently fabricate on the way to cowl the benefit or advantage received due to breaking a rule or said expectation.The man or woman who broke the curfew have come to be capable of stay at the birthday party for longer, whilst the simplest who drives too speedy is past due because of the truth he hit the snooze button on his alarm clock while it went off. If his lie is notion, the accomplice who says that he have grow to be "working" late in a resort room alongside with his lady friend even as the ringer at the mobile phone at his place of job should were switched off will not be held answerable for the results of his deception. In every one of these conditions, the individual that breaks the guideline makes the aware choice, previous to breaching the rule of thumb, that if faced approximately dishonest, they may lie to conceal their tracks. A excessive rating on an examination, for example, could have been acquired without cheating now and again;

but, this will no longer have been as easy and could have required greater artwork (hours of take a look at in this situation).

Keeping a person secure from capability risk

People make severe falsehoods for lots of motives, the second one maximum critical of this is to defend every exclusive character from capability risk. Even in case you disagree with what the character you are trying to guard did that positioned him or her in hazard, you continue to want to guard them because you do not want your friend, your coworker, your sister, your associate, or all of us else who you care approximately to be punished for some aspect they did. It isn't possible to mention for wonderful whether or not or not or not the majority of human beings aid those falsehoods. We apprehend the motivations of police officers who pick now not to testify toward a fellow officer who has broken the law; but, many humans accept as true with that law enforcement officials need to tell the reality.However, the names we supply them, which consist of rats, finks, and snitches, are pejorative. There are anonymous name-in lines to be had just so folks who offer information can also moreover shield their reputations and stay out of harm's way even as doing so. Do we keep people to a exquisite ultra-modern after they tell us when they do it of their very own will in preference to when they achieve this in reaction to a right away request to expose data? When I write in a later email on children's lying and the reasons why we do now not need children to tattle, I will take every distinct check this hassle and offer an explanation for why.

Self-Protection

One such reason can be which you need to prevent yourself from being damaged even when you have now not violated any pointers. The teen who's home by myself and responds to a traveller at the door by means of way of pronouncing, "My father is having a nap; come once more later," has now not completed a wrongdoing that they will be searching for to cowl up; instead, they'll be telling a lie to protect themselves.

Some human beings inform falsehoods that permits you to get the admiration of others. An obvious instance of this is bragging about a few aspect that isn't right. It is not unusual in children, or perhaps a few teens and adults had been observed to have it. If it seems to be actual, it will damage the boaster's reputation, but it may not do lots more than that. When a person makes a fraudulent declare approximately having made coins for beyond buyers, they're stepping into an unlawful arena.

Keeping one's privateness in tact

Another reason humans lie is to defend their privacy without without delay exercising their right to accomplish that.An example of this may be a daughter who responds to her mother's query, "who had been you speaking to at the cellular telephone simply now?" through pointing out her female buddy rather than the male who has virtually asked her out on a date. It is high-quality even as there can be a sturdy, trusting connection that a teen will feel ambitious sufficient to nation, "it in reality is private," as a end result proclaiming the right to have a secret. Only then will the child be given as authentic with they have got the right to preserve a mystery. Trust is going to be some other challenge I cover massive in upcoming troubles of my book.

The Exciting Adventure of It All!

Some people inform lies handiest for the leisure of seeing how a ways they are capable of push topics, exploring their hitherto untapped capability. A authentic big sort of kids, subsequently of their childhoods, should mislead their parents on cause just to check their limits and be aware if they will. Some humans interact on this behavior on a regular foundation due to the fact they admire the energy that contains controlling the facts that is to be had to the goal.

Avoiding Embarrassment

One in addition purpose human beings inform falsehoods, every crucial and little, is to shop themselves from disgrace. If the kid did no longer fear being punished for her failure and as an opportunity feared being embarrassed through manner of it, then one instance is probably the child who claimed that the wet seat turn out to be as a consequence of a damaged glass of water as opposed to the kid wetting her pants.

Keeping a low profile and defensive one's recognition are not unusual motivations for telling falsehoods that fall below the class of "lies of every day existence." People frequently inform lies that permits you to escape embarrassing or tough social conditions. It's feasible that they do now not comprehend the way to do it; as an excuse, they said that they "can't reap a babysitter" to interrupt out some special dull middle of the night and meal. "Sorry, I'm on my way out the door," an evidence provided with the aid of those who do not experience formidable enough to be honest, even to a very unknown cellphone shop clerk, is an example of a word that starts offevolved with "sorry" and ends with "on my way out."

Being Polite

Then there are the lies which is probably critical to hold polite social interplay, which embody "thank you very a top notch deal for the incredible party" or "that colour certainly appears nice on you." I do no longer be given as real with them to be falsehoods inside the same manner as bluffing in poker, performing in a play, or the asking charge no longer being the promoting fee are all examples of things that I regard as lies. There is usually a few form of be conscious, despite the fact that the intention does not expect being informed the reality in any of these conditions. However, the imposter is a liar, and so is the con artist, given that each of them take benefit of the reality that we've the expectation that the truth may be furnished to us. My next e-mail may have similarly statistics on the severa strategies of deception, along side this one.

Do we virtually need to find out whether a person has been lying to us?

In the majority of situations, there is no speedy or smooth approach to perceive dishonesty, or maybe if there were, we may not like what we studies despite the truth that we have been able to accumulate this.

Therefore, notwithstanding the fact that many humans say they're interested in reading the truth, there are various conditions wherein it's far lots less hard and greater great to really be given falsehoods. In the ones situations, we will be predisposed to push aside signs of dishonesty and make excuses for actions that could usually enhance suspicion for you to avoid the in all likelihood detrimental outcomes of discovering the falsehoods we were informed.

Chapter 8: Pathological Liars

Pathological liars utter falsehoods without any apparent purpose for their behavior. This type of deception is outstanding from nonpathological mendacity, in which the fib is frequently endorsed as it offers some kind of gain.

When people engage socially with one another, lying is a conduct that regularly happens. Certain animals, together with monkeys, have been visible engaging in this behavior.

There is a robust correlation among telling lies and gaining some income. For example, someone may furthermore lie to keep away from social disgrace. Although a few humans lie greater regularly than others, lying itself isn't always usually indicative of a intellectual fitness ailment, even though a few human beings lie greater often than others.

Lying pathologically is a separate difficulty. It's possible that this behavior is a symptom of a deeper mental health trouble, collectively with a individual disorder.

This page gives a higher communicate of pathological lying, together with a manner to discover the condition similarly to a manner to deal with the conduct of individuals who exhibit it.

What exactly is the pathology of mendacity?

When a person makes a fake statement with the purpose of misleading others, most usually for a few sort of personal advantage, this conduct is referred to as lying.

The sort of mendacity that does not imply a intellectual health state of affairs is known as nonpathological lying. Someone who suffers from pathological lying will inform falsehoods again and again, despite the fact that there is no obvious cause for them to carry out that.

There have been some efforts made to provide an reason of the variations among a pathological lie and a nonpathological lie, but further have a have a look at is needed to create appropriate variations a few of the varieties of lies.

One of the defining tendencies of a pathological lie is the absence of a smooth purpose for the deception. It is usually honest to decide why someone has informed a lie, which include to advantage themselves or to interrupt out an unpleasant or difficult social state of affairs. However, mendacity, it really is pathological, takes place for no apparent reason and does not appear to benefit the character.

It isn't appeared if a person who lies pathologically is aware about the dishonesty they're undertaking or whether or no longer they will be able to questioning sensibly approximately their lying behavior.

Lying to a pathological diploma can also make it hard to have interaction with exceptional people and can purpose big troubles in a single's relationships with loved ones and coworkers.

Causes

There hasn't been plenty have a look at achieved on this location, so the elements that result in pathological lying are though a mystery.

There is a loss of consensus on whether or no longer pathological mendacity is a sign of some other illness or a situation in and of itself.

For example, compulsive lying is a symptom of a number of distinctive illnesses, together with factitious problems and man or woman disorders.

Disturbance that isn't actual.

A sickness referred to as factitious illness, from time to time known as Munchausen's syndrome, is characterized by using the use of a person's conduct that indicates they may be affected by a intellectual or bodily contamination whilst in truth they may be no longer.

When one character falsely accuses some different of having an contamination, this conduct is called Munchausen's syndrome thru proxy. The substantial majority of times of this sickness are located in women of reproductive age who fake infection of their youngsters after which deceive clinical specialists approximately it.

There is not any smooth understanding of what motives factitious sickness. Among the hypotheses are:

For natural or genetic motives.

Abuse or forget about about throughout adolescence

A lack of vanity

A prognosis of a persona ailment is present.

Abuse of substances.

Despair

Disturbances of the persona

One of the ability signs of some character troubles is pathological mendacity. These personality problems embody:

BPD stands for borderline character ailment.

Narcissistic character disorder (NPD)

A sickness of the antisocial character (APD)

A man or woman who struggles with borderline character disease (BPD) might also moreover discover it hard to hold emotional control. People who be troubled through BPD regularly have excessive shifts in their mood, document better ranges of instability and absence of self belief, and do now not have a regular experience of who they're.

Characteristics of a narcissistic persona sickness encompass delusions of excellent significance in addition to an insatiable choice for adulation and preferential remedy.

Researchers contend that human beings with APD frequently lie for his or her private non-public advantage or entertainment, however the reality that human beings with this contamination are theoretically capable of mission pathological mendacity.

A individual who has borderline personality sickness (BPD) or non-borderline character contamination (NPD) may also want to inform lies if you need to twist reality into some detail this is greater constant with the feelings that they may be experiencing in location of the records.

These character problems also can result in huge problems in forming and maintaining connections with exceptional humans.

Frontotemporal dementia

According to the findings of a case have a take a look at done on a unmarried character displaying proof of pathological mendacity, the man or woman's behavioral styles were similar to the ones that could stand up with frontotemporal dementia.

Changes in behavior and language are signs and symptoms and signs and symptoms of frontotemporal dementia, a form of dementia that influences the frontal and temporal areas of the thoughts and is associated with age-associated cognitive decline.

These adjustments may also include the subsequent;

Irrelevant social conduct

Incapacity to empathize.

A diminishing functionality to apprehend one's non-public and distinct human beings's actions.

Alters in a single's tastes for wonderful food.

Obsessive and compulsive conduct

Boredom

Agitation

Indicators and manifestations

Lying is a compulsive conduct that might start on a small scale in pathological cases. It's viable for the falsehoods to often get extra complicated and dramatic over time, specifically if it's miles required to use them as a cowl for a preceding deception. They frequently come to be difficult to understand due to an excessive amount of superfluous fabric.

It isn't always normally the case that individuals who lie regularly also are pathological liars. One of the most defining traits of a pathological lie is the absence of any justification for the deception.

Therefore, a person who continuously ornaments tales so that you could make themselves appearance extra fascinating or who continuously lies that lets in you to cover up mistakes that they have made isn't probable to be a pathological liar for the reason that these behaviors aren't regular with pathological lying. These are apparent motivations that serve to further first-rate pastimes.

Lies of a pathological type are smooth for others to debunk, which may additionally additionally have a awful impact on the person that says them ultimately. For instance, the individual must stage baseless fees in competition to others or make outlandish assertions about their facts, every of which is probably clean for others to verify.

Diagnosis

It isn't always feasible to get a right evaluation for pathological mendacity; although, a physician or therapist may additionally moreover pick out out the conduct as an indication of each distinct hassle, which include a person sickness or factitious ailment, which may be the underlying reason.

These situations are characterized via the usage of overlapping signs and symptoms, one in every of this is the obsessive need to lie. People who're affected by those ailments additionally display off more symptoms.

Some people interact in pathological lying even inside the absence of some special underlying clinical hassle, which indicates that it's miles feasible for pathological lying to feature as its very very own impartial symptom.

Because there aren't any mental or herbal checks for it, diagnosing someone as having a pathological mendacity disease may be hard for scientific professionals.

A medical interview is what a physician will make use of to diagnose the big majority of intellectual health troubles. If the affected person isn't always coming near near about their lying, the attending medical doctor may want to are looking for recommendation from the affected person's loved ones or friends for assistance in recognizing the traits of pathological lying.

How to address a compulsive liar even as preserving your very very own integrity.

Dealing with a person who tells falsehoods on a pathological diploma can be quite hard. It also can moreover take some time and effort earlier than you may bring together a sincere reference to this individual and then keep it going.

It is important to preserve in thoughts that the person telling those falsehoods could not goal to do every body any harm or gain some issue from them. Lying pathologically may end up a compulsive conduct, and this behavior nearly constantly has excessive repercussions for the person who engages in it. Therefore, make an effort no longer to react violently or factor the finger of blame of their direction for the falsehoods.

It is useful to be aware that pathological mendacity may be an instance of an underlying highbrow fitness infection. Being privy to this truth is also beneficial. By asking the person whether or not or not or no longer they may be experiencing any extra signs and signs, you can assist them recognize the difficulty handy and determine whether or not or no longer to are seeking for recommendation from a therapist or a medical doctor for assist.

Treatment

Since pathological lying isn't an officially identified sickness, there may be no set therapy for it that can be observed.

If a medical medical doctor has motive to don't forget that the affected character's mendacity is the end result of an underlying ailment, they could advocate remedy for that situation.

For instance, the remedy for individual troubles often includes psychotherapy together with medicine.

Because pathological lying can also moreover furthermore motive damage to humans spherical the person that does it, a medical doctor may additionally suggest counseling for the individual's loved ones. They may have interplay with a therapist who will help them in dealing with the reactions that they have got to the problem.

Chapter 9: Methods For Discovering The Truth

1. Raise your diploma of self-popularity approximately the fact-based presumptions which you've been making. The majority of us bury our truth assumptions to this point down in our subconscious that we do now not even apprehend what it's far that we are supposing to be real. When the ones round us take delivery of as true with something to be real or whilst we have been "raised" to suppose a wonderful manner, we typically tend to embrace that belief as reality. That does now not advise that the aforementioned matters are, in truth, true. It's critical for us to make up our very very own minds, even though it is feasible that they will be right.

2. Recognize and appreciate the fact that many humans ought to have one-of-a-kind views on an entire lot of topics.These numerous elements of view aren't necessarily accurate or incorrect; instead,

they'll be just great. Everyone has the proper to have their non-public opinion, regardless of whether or not or not or now not or not it aligns with yours. Make an try and have an open thoughts and recognize the reasoning behind different factors of view.

3. Do not make hasty commitments to a specific element of view except you have were given given it careful thought.It is surely OK or maybe a top notch hassle as a way to check and understand the severa viewpoints on a subject, in addition to the reasons why one-of-a-type people may additionally have severa ideals, and to be conscious that this is the case. According to the terms of F. Scott Fitzgerald, "The take a look at of a brilliant thoughts is the capability to keep contradictory standards in the thoughts at the identical time, and but however keep the capability to carry out."

Four. If you want to comprehend a component of view that is not similar to yours, try and interest at the similarities in choice to the versions. What do the two of you seem to agree on?What shape of presumptions are the two of you making? Are you every strolling for some of the same dreams first of all, however then using extremely good tactics to get there? Are you both studying the equal strategies but coming to exceptional conclusions about the relative importance of the numerous additives that have to be taken into consideration? After locating out the parallels and differences, the opposing function will appear like the more low-price possibility. Even in case you keep to disagree, at least you may have a higher knowledge of the motives in your function.

5. Keep in thoughts that the manner terms are used and the emphasis placed on them are often the source of misunderstandings. It's no longer unusual to find out that you

and each different character are "in violent accord." You may additionally use a totally new language, or you may use the identical phrases however interpret them in a first rate manner. But in case you take some time to sincerely define what every of you is trying to specific, you can discover which you're in truth going for the identical intention.

6. When it involves vast subjects, you need to invite yourself those questions regarding the viewpoints of the man or woman talking or writing:

Does this make experience? Is it probably? The greater superb a few difficulty is, the more suspicion you want to have within the route of it. People will say outlandish topics because they understand that doing so gets them interest and maybe even land them a gap in the headlines. It is also more probable that outrageous claims may be repeated to distinctive people, with none shape of confirmation, of path.

Is it risky to the human beings spherical you? If that is the case, you owe it to those people, even in case you do no longer realize who they may be, to verify the statement in advance than you repeat it to wonderful humans.

Is there evidence to manual the declare being made? How do you recognise? Where did the purported records come from within the first location? Is it possible to depend on this supply? Where did the records that the supply supplied come from? Investigate the origins of the information to decide whether or not or no longer they're reliable.

If the statement isn't always primarily based totally on any information, then the character making the declaration is inquiring for that you agree with in them. Do you accept as true with you studied so? Do you've got any motive to place your faith in them? Is there any reason the speaker or creator should need to misinform you or "twist" the records in a manner this is more beneficial to themselves than to you?

Be on the lookout for emotionally charged phrases which includes "racist," "terrorist," "meltdown," "bailout," and other comparable terms that deliver more which means that to an obvious statement of reality. Whether you update the emotionally charged phrases with words that lack feeling or now not, you could test to look if the sentence however makes experience.

Keep an eye fixed fixed fixed out for overstatements that deliver some factor this is generally unremarkable an air of importance that it does no longer deserve (for instance, "A new have a look at indicates that half of of the arena's populace is beneath common").

Don't be duped thru numbers and probabilities. If some element isn't proper, which includes facts to it need to no longer make it greater truthful, especially if the figures are made up or if the data originates from a survey or studies this is biased. Verify in which the information came from, and inside the occasion that they had been gathered via a survey, take a look at to peer that the questions have been now not deliberately designed to misinform respondents (that may be a common tactic for manipulating the results of a survey), and that the sample length used inside the survey because it should be displays the population being surveyed.

Be cautious now not to confuse the concept of correlation with that of causation and impact. Even whilst one detail (as an example, poverty) is confirmed to have a correlation with each different detail (as an instance, weight troubles), this doesn't constantly endorse that the primary component causes the second aspect, nor does it entail that the second thing reasons the primary detail. Both of these variables may be the surrender end result of a few different problem. However, proponents of a certain thing of view may additionally employ data on this sort of manner as to offer the affect that there is a cause-and-impact hyperlink among matters while, in fact, there may be definitely a correlation.

7. Create a strong basis via compiling a listing of credible resources.When thinking about potential sources within the areas of politics, religion, and the media, it's miles important to bear in mind how one-of-a-kind humans see the ones regions. If a brilliant percent of people regard the facts you received from your supply as being excessive, you want to check whether or not or now not or no longer you must embody that facts on your base.

Eight. Utilize the property you have got got to be had to you as a "norm," and select the reliability of extra statistics resources primarily based definitely totally on how they range from your norm. Any statistics supply that extensively deviates from the norm which you frequently rely upon need to be subjected to in addition examination earlier than you get preserve of that new records supply as an exquisite one.

9. Try to preserve some consistency within the opinions you preserve. In the occasion that a information article takes a weird turn, together with positing a massive conspiracy principle, it must be known as into query. Your response want to be gradual and staged, together along with your mind-set regularly transferring as you acquire increasingly evidence to once more up the claims made inside the records. Be careful not to overreact.

10. If you really want to, you may label your self an extremist. You can be deemed an extremist if the data which you get from your property is likewise judged to be immoderate. But you must be aware that beliefs held via way of extremists are extensively remarkable from the ones held

by using the use of maximum human beings, that many people receive as actual with such perspectives to be incorrect, and that almost all of human beings regard the reviews held by means of the use of the use of extremists to lack credibility. If you want to have a better understanding of the mind held with the useful resource of the bulk of the populace, you want to recollect receiving a number of your facts and facts from extra mild resources.

Indications that the opposite celebration is lying

Did you understand that quality fifty 4% of folks that lie may be caught within the act? According to Vanessa Van Edwards, author of the primary splendid-promoting ebook inside the u . S . A . Titled Captivate in addition to the founder and critical investigator of the business enterprise called the Science of People, extroverts will be predisposed to lie more frequently than introverts do.

Her research determined that as a minimum eighty two percentage of falsehoods pass neglected, that is what inspired her to create a schooling utility within the art work of lie detection with the call "How to Be a Human Lie Detector." According to the findings of studies with the emerge as aware about "Prevalence of Lying in America," just six out of ten Americans claimed to talk the truth each day. These findings advise that taking this kind of path may be a worthwhile funding.

Given those information, a unmarried country's word, no matter the truth that it were to be sworn to underneath oath, might not be specifically dependable. Even if round 1/2 of the populace claims to be speaking the truth, there are certain strategies with the aid of which people might also beautify their functionality to encounter the fact if you want to guard themselves from emotional and financial disaster. The correct news is that there are some techniques that people can do this.

Despite the truth that lie detection education are beneficial for face-to-face encounters, the falsehoods that motive the greatest economic damage within the twenty first century are those which is probably communicated thru digital manner. According to USA.Gov, people can be duped or threatened to reveal their non-public information or financial assets using a whole lot of communication strategies, which includes the telephone, e mail, text messages, online advertisements, and social media.

How a first-rate deal in their private tough-earned coins have people out of region even as they were beneath duress? According to the Federal Trade Commission, sufferers of fraud referred to dropping a whopping $1.Forty eight billion in 2018, that may be a 38 percent growth over the previous one year's fashionable (FTC).

Adults of their 20s stated an average loss of $4 hundred in 2018, but parents in their 70s stated an average loss of $751 within the identical 3 hundred and sixty 5 days. And the sufferers aren't simply older people. People of their 80s, who misplaced a median of $1,seven hundred within the identical yr, observed that figure extra than quadruple to more than four,000.

Never, ever provide out your non-public information or ship cash by using using manner of cord transfer to someone you do not know a terrific way to guard your financial and personal property from liars. This piece of advice cannot be stressed sufficient.

It could not count number number whether or now not you are coping with faux internet threats or dishonest folks that misinform your face; the issue of the way to tell on the same time as a person is mendacity despite the fact that stands. According to Vanessa Van Edwards, doing so is one of the first activities in order to get familiar with the normal conduct of a person. This is the method of creating a baseline, which she describes as "how a person behaves at the same time as they'll be in ordinary, non-threatening conditions [...] Or how a person seems at the same time as they may be talking the reality." This is the way of installing area a baseline.

In one in all a type terms, it can be hard to determine while a person is lying in case you do now not recognize how they behave whilst they may be speaking the reality, which highlights the want to increase believe with someone in advance than you percentage personal information with them or reveal personal information with them. For instance, it's miles always excellent to call your economic corporation right now and apprehend who you are talking with as opposed to trusting someone who calls at random or sends an awesome-searching letter inside the mail claiming to be an employee of the financial institution. This is due to the truth random callers and letter senders are more likely to be scam artists.

On the alternative hand, if you understand a person and locate your self thinking whether or not or not you're being given the complete fact or a half of-fact, here is a list of the top 10 signs and symptoms that a person is mendacity this is sponsored up by means of the use of manner of clinical research.

1. A TRANSFORMATION IN SPEECH PATTERNS

Irregular speech styles are a red flag that a person won't be giving the general fact after they speak. According to a bit of writing that modified into published in Real Simple with the aid of Gregg mccrary, a former FBI criminal profiler, a person's voice or habits of talking may also moreover modify when they lie. Mccrary made the ones observations based totally on interviews that he carried out.

Mccrary begins via the use of the approach of figuring out a person's regular speech styles and mannerisms via asking popular, clear-cut inquiries, which incorporates what the man or woman's call is and in which they're dwelling. This permits mccrary to installation a baseline for studying the character's conduct. This offers him the ability to look any adjustments in speech or trends that could upward push up because of his asking greater hard and investigative inquiries.

2. The use of non-congruent gestures with the language

It is possible to decide whether or not or now not someone is mendacity with the useful resource of seeing whether or now not or no longer or now not they shake their head positive or no after answering fantastic. Non-congruent gestures are moves in the frame that don't healthful the phrases someone says, and the gestures are the truth-tellers, in step with Dr. Ellen Hendriksen, a scientific psychologist at Boston University's Center for Anxiety and Related Disorders, who became quoted in Scientific American. Dr. Hendriksen works at the Center for Anxiety and Related Disorders. According to the state of affairs provided with the useful resource of Dr. Hendricksen, if a person responds, "Of course i'll help with the inquiry," but then makes a hint head shake, there is a danger that they will no longer show the entire reality and no longer something but the fact for the duration of the studies.

3. Failure to Say Enough

When witnesses who are speaking the fact are puzzled extra approximately what they noticed and requested, "Is there something else?", new information are disclosed. But at the equal time as pressed to difficult on their prefabricated claims, liars offer subsequent to no greater statistics, if any the least bit.

People who, even as added on to reply questions or deliver additional details, often deliver a great deal much less information than folks which are talking the reality are referred to as "liars who lie by way of omission" by way of manner of researchers who're referenced inside the American Psychological Association (APA). This can be verified thru the usage of transcripts of telephone conversations or witness testimony, or it can be deduced from the reality that a discussion carries few descriptive phrases.

Asking members to retell what took place in reverse is each distinct method that researchers use to verify the reality. Truth-tellers will preserve to the identical story even as presenting more statistics, on the same time as liars will regularly get caught up in developing a separate story whilst not along with any information to the previous one. Truth-tellers will keep on with the same story on the identical time as supplying more statistics.

Four. EXPRESSION OF SELF

On the opportunity hand, researchers from Harvard Business School observed that those who are deliberately trying to find to mislead others stretch the reality thru the use of an excessive wide kind of terms. Because this shape of liar may additionally additionally make matters up as they pass alongside, they may moreover have a propensity to function too much detail so as to steer themselves or others of what they may be pronouncing. They might also upload phrases to the tale that a person who changed into imparting the truth can also in no manner have idea of in conjunction with.

Other language clues that were uncovered through this research demonstrated that liars had an inclination to use more profanity and zero.33-individual pronouns (alongside aspect he, she, and they) to take away themselves from any first-character participation (along with I, my, or mine).

Five. An Unusual Increase or Decrease in Vocal Tone

In the equal paper posted with the aid of the APA, a significant trouble is brought up about how detecting falsehoods is stricken by life-style, context, and communication.

When identifying whether or no longer or now not someone is mendacity, researchers want to preserve in thoughts cultural bias, in step with Dr. David Matsumoto, a professor of psychology at San Francisco State University and the CEO of Humintell, a consulting enterprise that trains human beings to check human emotions. Humintell trains people to observe facial expressions. His research on the detection of lies determined, for example, that Chinese people had a bent to speak with a higher voice pitch even as they are mendacity. Participants of Hispanic foundation within the studies take a look at, but, lied whilst speakme at a decrease voice pitch.

This examine demonstrates that non-verbal signs of lying can also correspond with cultural variations; subsequently, it is vital to take the ones versions into attention even as assessing others in area of relying surely on one's very very own cultural thoughts.

6. THEIR EYE DIRECTION

Truthfulness and making eye contact had been the subjects of severa communication nowadays. In the united states, there may be a cultural perception this is going a few thing like this: if someone isn't making eye touch, they are not talking the reality. However, in particular cultures, making eye contact is probably visible as untrustworthy relying at the times.

The speculation that humans gaze to the left or right even as they may be mendacity come to be rejected in studies that come to be posted in Plos One in 2012 and headlined "The Eyes Don't Have It." Nevertheless, regular with the findings of a research study that turn out to be performed in 2015 with the aid of the University of Michigan and published in Time Magazine, seventy percentage of individuals in a hundred and twenty media clips lied however preserving direct eye contact.

7. COVERING THEIR EYES OR MOUTH

It's feasible that many humans cowl their eyes or lips with their palms after telling a falsehood because of the reality they want to cowl their response to the deception or due to the fact they need to cover up the lie they just said. According to information which have grow to be furnished with the aid of former CIA operatives of their e-book titled "Spy the Lie," it has been observed out that once humans are mendacity, they

180

might even virtually close their eyes. This can be the case mainly at the equal time as it is in answer to a query that does not require a first rate deal of introspection at the a part of the respondent.

Eight. EXTREME FIDGETING

Imagine a infant being requested wherein the very last cookie went and what they may say in response. They may additionally additionally need to lick their lips, have a examine their fingernails, or maybe shake their palms earlier than mendacity about the most vital difficulty in the international.

According to the previous CIA dealers mentioned in Parade Magazine, what's occurring is that their tension reaction has kicked in, which motives blood to be evacuated from their extremities. This takes vicinity at the same time as humans experience threatened or disturbing. They may be subconsciously seeking to calm that tension response or at least get the blood flowing once more to their extremities, all of which can also hint at problem about talking a lie. It is also viable that they're looking for to get the blood flowing all over again to their extremities.

Nine. FINGER POINTING (LITERATURE OR IMAGERY)

According to Business Insider, the act of pointing in the course of or at a few factor or a person else, whether or not or not with the useful resource of gestures or words, may moreover signify an unmistakable motive to shift interest far from someone and placed the obligation for the state of affairs on a person else.

Having a baseline facts of whether or now not or not that individual often uses gesticulation or finger pointing frequently might be beneficial, of course. On the alternative hand, if a person has a peaceful and gathered way of speech in place of an hostile one which consists of pointing palms, this aggressive flip can be an illustration that a person is lying.

10. Confessing one's personal reputation as a "GOOD LIAR"

Allow the liar to talk for you. This is probable the simplest approach to figuring out a liar. Research that grow to be completed in 2019 and published in Plos One beneath the become aware about "Lie occurrence, lie features, and methods of self-reported superb liars" demonstrated that folks who self-pick out as "suitable liars" are a higher honest indication than lie detector tests.

According to the findings of this research, "unique liars" commonly endorsed white lies to their coworkers and friends face-to-face and concentrated on handing over recollections which have been honest and clean to recognize. One smooth lesson that may be drawn from this take a look at is that you need to not placed your faith in someone who brags about being a expert liar.

www.ingramcontent.com/pod-product-compliance
Lightning Source LLC
Chambersburg PA
CBHW062141020426
42335CB00013B/1287